# Frazzled, Fried...Finished?
# A Guide to Help Nurses Find Balance

Borgatti Communications
www.joanborgatti.com
2004

# Frazzled, Fried...Finished?
# A Guide to Help Nurses Find Balance

Joan C. Borgatti, RN, MEd

## Also by Joan Borgatti

*Because I Can*

# Acknowledgements

My path of exploration and discovery has included twisted turns and difficult terrain that I managed to travel, until finally a more welcoming path revealed itself to me. Many people appeared just when I needed them, while others disappeared or disappointed. Either way, I learned so much from all of you.

I'm grateful to my family. You offered me food when I forgot to eat, solace and support when my computer plotted against me, and the belief that I could finally complete this book.

Many grateful thanks to Kerri Richardson, talented editor and compassionate coach and friend, who convinced me to write this book. You always know just what to say to push me beyond my innate laziness!

Thanks to Karla Knight, writer and friend, who provided the opportunity that inspired me to write this book. I so appreciate our coffee get-togethers!

And finally, I want to say 'thank-you' to all the nurses in the trenches of healthcare. You are the inspiration for this book. And you are heroes, one and all.

# Table of Contents

# Introduction

I fell into nursing. At least that's what it felt like at the time. When I was a little girl growing up in the 1950's, I never thought about becoming a nurse. My dreams included writing the Great American Novel. But somehow I fell into nursing and fell in love with the profession.

When I say I fell into nursing, I'm not kidding. Finding my career was just one of the many examples in my life where it seemed I was guided by a force far more intelligent than I could ever be.

Example number one: When I was just at the point of 'considering the possibility' of a nursing career, I called a school of nursing to request a catalog. But fateful forces were at work behind my back again. Somehow, my call was accidentally diverted and I found myself on the phone with the dean of the school of nursing. I quickly panicked and explained that I was merely calling for a catalog. She seemed not to hear me and explained that she had one more "slot" to fill for the upcoming class the following month, and she wanted to meet me face-to-face for an interview. You've got the picture. I was sitting in that nursing class before the catalog hit my doorstep!

I found that I loved nursing and quickly became passionate about the career. The rest, as they say, is history. After the requisite time in med/surg I moved on to pediatrics in an acute care setting, did some utilization review, and then practiced as a school nurse for a K-4 elementary school. I learned so much in every practice area. Everywhere I worked there were extraordinary men and women who exemplified the best of nursing, and earned my awe and star-struck admiration every day.

But my passion for writing was also large. Was there a way to blend the two passions? Happily, yes. This leads me to example number two: I strongly felt that there was a way to blend nursing and writing. So guided by an inner gut feeling, I took a year-long leave of absence from my position as a school nurse. I started journaling faithfully every day, describing what I envisioned as the perfect job. I even wrote in my journal where I would like the job to be located. To make a long story short, I applied for a blind ad in the newspaper looking for an RN/Editor. Hmmm....I thought, I'm not an editor but I do write. I applied and was invited to interview at a nearby hotel. The interview and subsequent interviews were unlike any I had ever experienced. The position was for a nursing magazine and the company did not want competition to realize that they were moving into my geographical area. So, I interviewed and eventually accepted the position of editor without ever seeing the magazine, knowing the name of the company, or knowing where my office would be located! Amazingly the office turned out to be located near the area that I had written in my journal as an ideal spot. Nevertheless, my husband thought I was absolutely out of my mind to accept such a strange job offer.

But my faithful guiding force and intuition told me to take the job. I held the position of editor and editorial director for nearly seven years and was fortunate to expand on my passion for writing and nursing. In that role I met and talked with nurses around the country and forever reinforced my belief that nurses are extraordinary and far too humble. It became increasingly important to me to help nurses see themselves in a realistic light and shed, once and for all, the mantle of humility I believe holds the profession back.

An example of just how nurses belittle themselves occurred early on in my nursing career when I "floated" to the ICU. The nurses in that unit were incredibly skilled and generously shared their knowledge with the novice – me! One of the patients needed to be transferred to a large hospital ICU and a nurse I particularly admired was assigned to monitor the patient in the ambulance during the transfer. I saw the nurse remove her scrub jacket that identified her as an ICU nurse and replace it with an unmarked jacket.

"Why did you change jackets?" I asked. She replied that she didn't want the "city" ICU nurses to look down at her because she practiced in a smaller hospital's ICU. In that one striking moment, I saw an ICU nurse with years of critical care experience shed her confidence as easily as she changed jackets. It's a moment and an image I never forgot. Scenes like that continue to play out in hospitals and healthcare settings, as nurses devalue who they are and what they know.

I've practiced in the healthcare trenches. Now that I no longer practice and have some distance from the battlefield, I can honestly say that I am even more in awe of what you do everyday in your practice. There are few certainties in life – certainly death and taxes come to mind. But one other certainty is that nurses are incredible people who deserve the respect, admiration, and compensation of the facilities they work for and the communities they serve.

There are few professions I admire more than nursing. Nurses are can-do people. No problem's too big; no emergency too large; no situation too immense. No matter the circumstances, nurses step up to the plate and get the job done with expert skills and enormous compassion.

It's quite possible that nursing is one of the most underrated and misunderstood professions. The public adores nurses, but they just don't 'get' that nursing is a complex and demanding profession that exacts a toll on every nurse who gives patient care his or her all.

And surprisingly, I think that sometimes nurses don't get it either. Nurses don't get how extraordinary they are, or all they bring to their practice. Instead, they run at full speed trying to do all that's asked of them and then some. So much so that they don't have time to catch their collective breath, look at what they've accomplished, and the depth of the impact they have on people's lives.

Here we sit, in the middle of a severe nursing shortage, as many exhausted and burned-out nurses struggle to make it from one shift to the next. Where did the idealism go? When did the hopes so many nurses started out with disappear? And more importantly, how can nurses find it again?

This book is aimed at helping you stop and take a moment to check in with yourself, figure out who you are and what you want, and hopefully rekindle the passion you once had. But you can't do that if the proverbial well is dry. You can't give and give and expect that your life will remain on track and run smoothly.

So a little coaching is in order. What's coaching, you ask? It is a partnership between a coach and a client that is directed at taking action-oriented steps toward what you want and away from what you don't want. It's as simple as that. A coach is someone who is always in your corner, cheering, supporting, and motivating you toward success.

Coaches in the athletic world are nothing new. But life coaching is a relatively new profession that helps clients focus on what is, not on what was. It's not therapy, and it's not grounded in the past. The focus is on the here and now. Coaches ask provocative questions and encourage clients to take the steps needed to get them where they want to go. And like an athletic coach, a life coach holds the client accountable.

This book is a coaching book just for nurses. It doesn't matter where you practice – in a hospital, school, business, or patient's home. The book is filled with strategies and tools to help you find balance between the demands of your professional life and your personal life. Do you need to set better boundaries? See chapter five. Is the clutter in your life out of control? See chapter three. Are you dealing with caring for children and your parents? See chapter two. Leadership, success, developing a vision, and giving a speech are just some of the topics addressed in this book. Of course, this book is not meant to be comprehensive. To fully benefit from a coaching experience, I recommended that you work with a coach one-on-one or in a small group.

Important to note, the purpose of this book is not to finger-point and blame healthcare facilities, administrators, or nonnurse colleagues for the negative experiences you might have had during the course of your career. That's not fair and it certainly does not consider your accountability and responsibility. So it's always a worthwhile exercise to ask yourself, What is my role in this? How do I figure in this outcome? Not only is it the responsible thing to do, it's also an important part of assessing who you are and how you can manifest the best possible outcome.

I know how busy you are. So use this book in whatever way makes sense for you. Start at the beginning and do the exercises as you go along, or skip to chapters that address a problem or issue that hits home for you.

It's your time now; it's your turn. It's time to step to the front of the line and administer a little TLC to yourself for a change. Enjoy the journey!

# About the Author

Joan C. Borgatti, RN, MEd, is an author, motivational speaker, and life coach. She is also the author of *Because I Can*. Hundreds of Joan's articles have appeared in regional and national publications, and she is a popular speaker on writing, life balance, and the nursing profession. She is the former editor and editorial director of a nursing magazine.

Her work has been covered by the media, and has included interviews in newspapers and on talk radio, such as *Defining Women* on WMRD (1150 AM). Joan has also been quoted in a number of publications, including the best-selling book, *Your Career: How to Make It Happen*.

Joan lives with her family outside Boston.

For more information about Joan's speaking, writing, or coaching, please contact:

Borgatti Communications
Website: www.joanborgatti.com
E-mail: coachborgatti@aol.com

Cover photo: Gretje Ferguson Photography
Image by Lori Johnson, Your Best Image

# Chapter One

## Assessment 101

"Learn to get in touch with silence within yourself and know that everything in this life has a purpose. There are no mistakes, no coincidences, all events are blessings given to us to learn from."

Elizabeth Kubler-Ross

What makes you tick? What drives your actions or is the cause of your inaction?

It's human nature to wonder why we do the things we do and think the way we think. Many times our needs drive our actions as we continuously play out, consciously and subconsciously, strategies to get those needs met once and for all.

Many of us live lives that don't even come close to meeting our personal requirements because we don't take the time to figure out what values, experiences, and things really feed our souls and make us happy.

Then there are the things in our life that drag us down and hold us back – tolerations. These are the things or people in our lives that drain our energy and annoy us, yet we seem powerless to address them.

In this chapter, we'll take a look at needs, requirements, and tolerations, and how to understand what they are and how to make them work for you in your life. It's all about doing a careful assessment; similar to the assessment you make when a new patient is admitted to your floor – What does this patient need? What care will this patient require? And what needs to be eliminated and prioritized to provide the best outcome for this patient?

The late Thomas Leonard, founder of Coach University and Coachville, explored the idea of needs, requirements, and tolerations, and his work has become the touchstone for coaching. And it's a great place to start.

### Needs

We all have basic human needs for clothing, shelter, food, and water. Those primary needs are not an option; they must be met. The same is true of other

1

needs we have that are specific to every human being. Though we probably won't die from not having a personal need met, we will not live the life that is most fulfilling to us and will always feel that there is a huge void in our lives.

For instance, you might have a need for order in your life. If things are not in the right place or some aspect of your life becomes chaotic, you are miserable and nothing seems to go right. On the other hand, your colleague has no such need for order and a messy nurse's station doesn't faze her a bit. But you can't even gather your thoughts and see beyond the mass of paperwork and discarded coffee cups.

We all have many needs, most of which are not met because we don't identify them and then make them a must in our lives. We don't yet see the value and the positive outcomes of making our needs a priority.

Take a look at Julie. Julie's a staff nurse who always seems to be patting herself on the back for everything she does. Sometimes the staff gets irritated with her constant need for approval and her sullen behavior when she isn't rewarded. People talk about how needy she is, and wonder why can't she just do her job and forget about bringing it to everyone's attention? The truth is, Julie *is* 'needy.' Her need for approval and acknowledgement is not being met in her professional life, and could be a result of her need not being met in her personal life as well.

Julie's need for approval and acknowledgement is driving her behavior. The good news is that if Julie is able to recognize that need and address it once and for all, it will no longer be a need in her life and will no longer drive her behavior. If Julie never reaches an understanding of how that need is driving her behavior and dominating her thoughts, she will continue to drive people away and continue the cycle.

And that's what our needs are all about: identifying our personal needs and modifying our behavior to get those needs met, rather than using behavior that only sabotages and prevents us from ever meeting those needs.

It's important to understand the genesis of that personal need. Is it an unmet need from childhood, for instance? Understanding where the need came from and why is an important way to honor and respect that need. Sometimes the source of the need is rooted deeply and is best addressed with therapy.

Your unmet needs are responsible in part for who you are as a person today. We are who we are as much by what needs we had met, as unmet. If you look closely at each unmet need, you will see a positive aspect that grew as a result of it.

Let's look at Julie again. Her unmet need for acknowledgment and approval causes her to always push herself to do more in her efforts to be noticed.

Consequently, her abilities as a staff nurse are impressive and she has often gone out of her way to learn new skills.

It's time to identify some of your needs. Read through the list of 200 needs below and circle ten words that resonate with you. Remember, needs are something you must have in your life to be your best. Take the time to really try on each word for size. Does it ring true for you? Also bear in mind that you may feel resistant about circling a word because you don't want it to be a personal need. It may be a need you're reluctant to acknowledge.

| **BE ACCEPTED** | **BE ACKNOWLEDGED** | **BE RIGHT** |
|---|---|---|
| Approved | Worthy | Correct |
| Included | Praised | Not mistaken |
| Respected | Honored | Honest |
| Permitted | Flattered | Morally right |
| Popular | Complimented | Deferred to |
| Sanctioned | Prized | Confirmed |
| Cool | Appreciated | Advocated |
| Allowed | Valued | Encouraged |
| Tolerated | Thanked | Understood |

| **TO ACCOMPLISH** | **BE LOVED** | **BE CARED FOR** |
|---|---|---|
| Achieve | Liked | Get attention |
| Fulfill | Cherished | Helped |
| Realize | Esteemed | Cared about |
| Reach | Held fondly | Saved |
| Profit | Desired | Attended to |
| Attain | Preferred | Treasured |
| Yield | Relished | Treated with tenderness |
| Consummate | Adored | Given gifts |
| Win | Touched | Embraced |

| **CERTAINTY** | **TO CONTROL** | **BE FREE** |
|---|---|---|
| Clarity | Dominate | Unrestricted |
| Accuracy | Command | Privileged |
| Assurance | Restrain | Immune |
| Obviousness | Manage | Independent |
| Guarantees | Correct others | Autonomous |
| Promises | Be obeyed | Sovereign |
| Commitments | Not be ignored | Not obligated |

Exactness
Precision

**BE COMFORTABLE**
Luxury
Opulence
Excess
Prosperity
Indulgence
Abundance
Not work
Taken care of
Served

**TO COMMUNICATE**
Be heard
Tell stories
Make a point
Share
Talk
Be listened to
Comment
Be informed
Advise

**PEACE**
Quietness
Calmness
Unity
Reconciliation
Stillness
Balance
Agreement
Respite
Steadiness

**POWER**
Authority
Capacity

Keep status quo
Restrict

**BE NEEDED**
Improve others
Be a critical link
Be useful
Be craved
Please others
Affect others
Give
Be important
Be material

**DUTY**
Be obligated
Do the right thing
Follow
Obey
Have a task
Satisfy others
Prove self
Be devoted
Have a cause

**RECOGNITION**
Be noticed
Be remembered
Be known for
Well regarded
Given credit
Acclaimed
Heeded
Seen
Celebrated

**SAFETY**
Secure
Protected

Self-reliant
Liberated

**HONESTY**
Forthrightness
Uprightness
Truthfulness
Sincerity
Loyalty
Frankness
Nonscheming
Directness
Candor

**ORDER**
Perfection
Symmetry
Consistency
Sequentially
Checklists
Unvarying
Rightness
Literalness
Regulated

**WORK**
Career
Performance
Vocation
Determination
Initiative
Tasks
Responsibility
Industriousness
Busyness

| | |
|---|---|
| Results | Stable |
| Omnipotence | Fully informed |
| Strength | Deliberate |
| Might | Vigilant |
| Stamina | Cautious |
| Prerogative | Alert |
| Influence | Guarded |

Now narrow your list of ten needs down to the four most important to you:

1. _____
2. _____
3. _____
4. _____

Now select just one of the four needs:
My chosen need to start working on is

_____

What is keeping you from getting that need satisfied now?

_____
_____
_____
_____
_____

Take action! What is one action step you can take today toward getting this need met? For instance, if you have a need to feel acknowledged you might want to share with loved ones that you would like some help meeting this need. It might go something like this, "I'd like your help getting this need met. So, it would be helpful if you could let me know when I've done something well. And, I'd be happy to do that for you as well."

When you've satisfied that need and you feel it is no longer a driving need for you, you can then move ahead with another need.

Julie grew tired of not getting her need for acknowledgement and approval met, and lonely because she seemed to push away the very people – colleagues, friends, and family – she wanted around her. She looked at the list of 200 needs and narrowed her list down to one primary need – to be valued.

To get that need met for her, Julie knew that she would need to take a risk and ask for what she needed. Here are a few things she did:

1. Modified her behavior. Julie knew her behavior was not helping her get her need met, and instead was pushing people away. She made a point of making sure that she genuinely praised other people for a job well done and cut down the number of times she sought approval.

2. Spoke candidly at a staff meeting and apologized if she had bothered anyone with her approval-seeking behavior. "For whatever reason, I need to feel that I am a valued member of this staff, and I don't feel it," said Julie. "I would appreciate it if you would all let me know when I've contributed in some way, and I will promise to do the same for you. I think this would really help me get this need met once and for all!"

## Requirements

Do you often wish people would treat you the way you want them to? And are you often surprised that people in your life don't know what you want? They should just know, you think. Rather than share your discontent, you withdraw or complain or just whine.

Don't confuse requirement with preference. A requirement is absolutely needed to make you feel satisfied. A preference would be nice, but it isn't an absolute necessity. When a preference is not met, it's not a huge deal. But when a requirement isn't met, you are likely to be upset.

Making other people – whether it's our work colleagues, loved ones, or people who provide services to us – aware of what we require doesn't just benefit us. It benefits the people we have enlightened, because it makes their lives so much easier. For instance, you're not happy with the way the drycleaner presses your suit, yet you're reluctant to let him know that you're not happy with the end result. Shouldn't he know how the suit should be done? After all, that's his business. So, you forget about it until the next time your suit is pressed and again find that it's just not what you want.

You have three choices: 1) Hope that the drycleaner figures out how you want the suit done and just deal with it when he doesn't, and continue to be upset. 2) Go to another drycleaner. 3) Let him know (in a respectful manner, of course) that the suit is not pressed to your liking and specify how you would like it to be done. You might say, "Mr. Smith, you always do such a wonderful job on all my drycleaning. And I'm sure you would want to know if I wasn't completely satisfied. I would prefer that you press my suit by

_____."

The problem with the first choice is that you are not informing others how you want to be treated or what you require (in this case, your suit pressed a certain way). Your dissatisfaction continues, your self-esteem plummets because you can't make your needs known, and your drycleaner remains clueless about how to best meet your service needs.

The second choice is just a way to escape out the back door, requires energy on your part, and never deals with your unrest head on. Choice #3 is the best choice because it lets your drycleaner know how to best serve you, which is what most business people would prefer rather than lose a customer, and it boosts your self-esteem because you voiced your requirements in that customer relationship.

Take a moment. What areas in your life are you not being specific about your requirements? If you need it, use a separate piece of paper.

_____
_____
_____
_____
_____
_____

What could you say to address the situation and get your requirements met?

_____
_____
_____
_____
_____

By making your requirements known, how would that make you feel? How would it impact the quality of your life?

_____
_____
_____

---
---
---

Giving people an opportunity to please you is really not difficult. In fact, it often takes the guessing out of the situation, which makes it much more pleasant for everyone. When we don't let people know how to meet our requirements, we become resentful and the situation can become much more of a problem as we find ourselves overreacting. And that's not fair to the people in our lives.

**Tolerations**

They can be the little things in our life that annoy us, or the big things in our life that are just a pain in the neck. Tolerations – those things that sap our energy, pull us down, and hold us back. We are surrounded by tolerations in our homes, in the workplace, and in our relationships.

Tolerations can include a backlog of bills that should be paid, the dentist appointment you've been meaning to make, the walls that need painting, the e-mail you've been meaning to respond to, or that presentation you keep putting off. In other words, anything that hangs over your head like an ominous cloud is a toleration that needs to be addressed and dealt with. Once the tolerations are cleared up, you will experience a surge of positive energy and you'll create space in your life for even greater things. This is because our mind doesn't have that negative energy hanging over us any longer. We're free! Well, almost.

Let's look at an example.

Kerri is a new nurse manager. Her desk looks like a cyclone hit it. She's got scheduling to do, a report to complete, a presentation to create, and she can't put her fingers on anything. Kerri prides herself on being a very "hands-on" manager, helping out on the floors when needed – which is often. A couple of staff nurses have already approached Kerri about vacation requests they submitted and there are rumblings about the schedule. Kerri feels as if a huge cloud follows her wherever she goes. Her tolerations include clutter and chaos, and until those are cleared up, she will continue to have rumblings from the staff nurses. She's let tolerations get the best of her, and it's keeping her from doing her job.

What can Kerri do? First, she needs to recognize the tolerations in her life – clutter, chaos, and procrastination – and begin to tackle them.

Kerri made a quick list of absolute must-do items. Here's how her list looks:

1. Scheduling. Must plug the holes and make sure staffing is okay first.

2. Clutter on desk. Need to organize files and get a handle on everything. Tell the staff I can't help out for a while until I have things under control.

3. Prepare my presentation. The presentation is due in two weeks, so I can't procrastinate any longer. Besides, I'll feel much better when that's done and ready to go.

4. Clear up vacation requests. Put process into place so this doesn't happen again. Make a 'tickler' note in my planner well before the summer to make sure vacation requests are in so I have more time to get coverage.

5. Complete report. Make sure I keep copies in a file so that it's easier to do report next time.

Now that Kerri has eliminated her tolerations, she finds that her office is neater, and she can put her hands on exactly what she's looking for. Instead of sighing when she enters her office, she now relaxes a bit and feels energetic enough to tackle whatever problems arise. Kerri notices that the staff seem more relaxed as well, and she believes it is because she's able to address their needs more easily. And while there will always be problems that arise, such as last-minute scheduling problems, Kerri believes she is ready to tackle them – one at a time.

Dealing with tolerations is best done head on. Identify what the toleration is and then chunk it down – break down the project into steps. Just taking an action toward eliminating a toleration will energize you.

It's your turn. Make a list of some things you are tolerating in your life. Use a separate piece of paper if you would like to add more categories or expand on them.

Your home.
   1._____
   2._____
   3._____
   4._____

Your family.
   1._____

2._____
3._____
4._____

Your friendships.

1._____
2._____
3._____
4._____

Your workplace.

1._____
2._____
3._____
4._____

Your career.

1._____
2._____
3._____
4._____

Now that you've identified some of your tolerations, go back and make a note of how you plan to eliminate each toleration. For instance, if one toleration is a feeling that your friendships are withering due to lack of attention, you might consider sharing that thought with your friends and your desire not to let that happen, or open your planner and schedule some get-togethers with your friends. Or perhaps you have been tolerating a long and stress-filled commute to work every day. Some strategies for eliminating that toleration might include 1) carpooling so that you have company on the commute, 2) if available, consider public transportation, 3) while driving, listen to books on tape, or 4) consider finding a healthcare facility closer to where you live.

Simply taking small steps will make an enormous difference in how you feel and your sense of control over your life.

# Resources

Leonard, T. *The Portable Coach*. Scribner. New York, NY:1998.

# Chapter Two

# CPR for Burnout

"You can get lonesome – being that busy."
Isabel Lennart

Nursing and burnout seem to go together. And it seems that nurses have been talking about burnout for as long as anyone can remember. You all know nurses who have left the profession because of burnout, or transferred to less demanding (is there such a thing?) practice areas.

But alas, it seems nurses moan and complain about the profession and how helpless they are to stem the tide of even more burnout. You've waited for it to pass, and guess what? It hasn't. So, maybe, just maybe, you need to take action to prevent burnout in the first place.

Some of the reasons for burnout include the demands on our personal lives. We're being pulled in many different directions. Other reasons include toxic relationships (see more about toxic work environments in chapter five) and the legacy we may be leaving behind by the continued abuse (yes, abuse) of the young nurses who are entering the profession.

Ready to perform CPR on your burnout? Look, listen, and feel.

## Sandwich Generation©

People are living longer. The baby boomers are aging. Welcome to the Sandwich Generation© – those who are still raising families and caring for parents. You're caught between two generations, and undoubtedly stressed by the demands you face. You have allegiance to those who raised you and an obligation to those you are still raising. That's a lot of stress and hard work, especially for nurses who often find themselves in the caretaker role at home and at work.

Oftentimes it seems that the role of caretaker for the older generation falls to the nurse in the family. Usually, it's the nurse who bears the weight of most, if not all, of the responsibility of caring for aging parents. The reasons that are floated about by other members of the family might include:

- I have a job. I can't just take time off from work to care for dear old Dad. (*Hmmm...that's funny, I thought my career as a nurse was a job. What was I thinking?*)

- I have bills and financial obligations to support my family. (*Oh, and my imaginary trust fund takes care of all my financial obligations and bills?*)

- I just don't have the time to care for Dad. (*Let me check my planner. What a surprise, it's full.*)

Ideally, everyone should have candid conversations with siblings and parents about how caretaking will look when the time arrives. Such a conversation allows parents to share how they would like to be cared for in their golden years, how they would prefer to maintain their independence, and how they financially want to prepare for it. This is the time when siblings can understand that this is a shared role, and understand their part in that role.

Unfortunately, it often doesn't work that way. It's true that the nurses in the family bring special skills and knowledge to the table. Nevertheless, that doesn't mean that those special skills and knowledge wipe the slate clean of responsibilities that other family members might have in sharing the caretaking of aging parents.

If you find yourself unfairly stuck between two generations of caretaking and lack the support of other family members – especially siblings – then some negotiating needs to be done.

Here are some things to consider:

- Siblings who are unable to help because they live too far away can provide financial support. This could mean money that would pay for respite or adult day care so that you could have free time to yourself.

- Siblings who live closer could share in the caretaking. If, for instance, they complain that a full-time job prevents them from helping out, it's only fair that they care for Mom or Dad on the weekends.

- Perhaps Mom or Dad could pay you for your time in caring for them, or their will could be amended to reflect the value of what you are doing. This may seem callous, but what it would allow is the opportunity for you to be compensated for your time and expertise and allow you to afford self-care to keep yourself from suffering from too much stress.

Dealing with siblings who leave the bulk, if not all, of responsibilities on your shoulders is unfair and thoughtless. That type of behavior sends a clear message that your needs fall far short of their needs. And it's possible that that behavior is a pattern that has played out in the past, and is not new.

But that doesn't mean you have to accept it. Setting firm and strong boundaries is an important tool for dealing with the burnout of being the sole caretaker of a parent. Hopefully, it's a tool that you can put into place before a situation like this arises. For more information on setting boundaries, see chapter five.

Carol Abaya is a journalist who has written frequently about the Sandwich Generation©. In fact, she is credited with coining the term and the concept. Here is her list of ten must-do steps for caring for an elder:

1.  Identify the people who should be involved. Meet in person, if possible, or have conference calls. (Note I've said calls, plural). Each person will undoubtedly bring different ideas, thoughts, and feelings to the table.

2.  Accept what is – the reality of your father's incapacity, your mother's seeming helplessness, your role reversal challenge.

3.  Identify goals. What are the clear needs of both parents?

4.  Discuss with your mother her feelings and identify what she really can and should do for herself. Encourage and help her to do more.

5.  Establish an ongoing dialogue with your father's doctors as to prognosis and care needs.

6.  Identify care alternatives and how they can best be handled. If finances and house space allow, can he be cared for at home with live-in, 24-hour help? Will he be better cared for in a nursing home – possibly with privately hired supplemental help?

7. Develop two care plans – one for your father and one for your mother. Keep them flexible and change as appropriate.

8. Divide chores between family members and seek other help resources.

9. Keep up the family dialogue and develop new ways of handling the situation as circumstances and needs change.

10. Don't carve in stone what should be done. Change is the name of the game.

With permission of Carol Abaya, The Sandwich Generation.com.

Being sandwiched between the demands of two generations can take its toll even under the most ideal of circumstances. Even the best of people – and nurses – become burned out in such situations. Develop a care plan for you. What outcome do you want? What steps can you put into place to make the situation easier for you to bear? What steps can you put into place to take better care of yourself and recharge your batteries? Are there community resources that could provide assistance? Check into your community Council on Aging, Meals on Wheels, adult day care programs, and so forth. Are there support groups for people also caring for aging parents? And don't forget to assess the impact of your stress level and caring for aging parents on your children. Provide regular opportunities for your children to share their feelings, too.

Take a few moments and start to line up your resources.

1. I need to talk to

_____

_____

2. I have been avoiding

_____

_____

3. My next step is

_____

_____

4. Resources available to me in the community are (if you don't know, that's your next step)

_____

_____

_____

_____

_____

There are valuable lessons in caring for aging parents – paying them in kind for caring for you all those years, and teaching your children, by example, how to respect and care for elders. But those lessons should not come at the expense of your physical or mental health.

Think about the following tips for finding moments to rejuvenate you:
- Get a massage.
- Have a standing date with your spouse to keep the relationship alive and flourishing.
- Sit in your local bookstore or library and soak up the silence and a good read.
- Take a walk.
- Make your physical health a priority – eat well and exercise.
- Talk to a good friend; one who gives you good advice.
- Take a long, hot bubble bath every evening to help decompress from the day.
- Do something silly and fun on a regular basis.

Take a moment and develop a care plan for taking care of you.
I understand that if I don't take care of myself I can't take care of anybody else.
I will take care of myself on a regular basis by:

_____

_____

_____

_____

_____

_____

## Toxic Relationships

You're giving report to the oncoming shift and have to stop every few sentences until Susan finishes giving her opinion on every aspect of patient care and her take on the patient's personality. You note the eyes rolling around you and you grit your teeth and try to get through report. Susan is oblivious to the eye rolling of her colleagues and your obvious displeasure. You note to yourself how different report is when Susan is off – everyone chats easily and the report just flows quickly. But when Susan's on, it's like the air is sucked right out of the room.

You've been 'friends' with Allison for years. But the relationship has never been easy. You always feel guarded and cautious about what you say. And countless times you've wondered why Allison "accidentally" let a confidence slip or embarrassed you in front of other people. She is always apologetic or innocently denies trying to hurt or embarrass you. You can't put your finger on it, but being with Allison always leaves you feeling like you're lacking something or that you're not good enough. But for the life of you, you don't know why.

You try your darndest, but your mother-in-law always finds a way to put you down. Your house isn't clean enough, your kids not smart enough, and your husband not happy enough. And she uses her other daughter-in-law as the poster child for perfect people. Try as hard as you might, you just can't seem to please her. You wonder, what am I doing wrong?

What do Susan, Allison, and your mother-in-law have in common? They are toxic to you. Interactions with them leave you feeling less than who you are. You are suffering from overdoses of toxic relationships, and it can be deadly – to your sense of self, physical well-being, and mental health.

It's not that Susan, Allison, or your mother-in-law are necessarily bad people. It's just that the chemistry is not right. In the case of Susan, it may be that her personality rubs you the wrong way, or that on some subconscious level she reminds you of an aspect of your own personality that you don't like. So, whenever Susan is around, you feel out of sorts and irritated by her. In the case of Allison and your mother-in-law, most likely it is a case of them not liking you, or some aspect of who you are. Either way, the relationships are toxic to you.

What do you do about toxic relationships? If someone in your life – be it a coworker, friend, or relative – is toxic to you, the best thing you can do is walk away from the relationship. Granted, this is not always possible.

Consider the case of the 'friend' Allison. Perhaps the first thing you need to do is examine your definition of friend and remember that a friend is someone who supports and champions you, even when you don't believe in yourself. A real friend does not make you feel like you are lacking in some aspect of your life, nor betray your confidences. This may be the time when walking away from the relationship is the best course of action. Here's how you might do that:

"Allison, I feel that our friendship has run its course. I want the best for you and I no longer feel that I can bring that to the friendship. I hope you understand."

This is a graceful way to end a friendship because it doesn't attack Allison. It just states how you feel. That is not to say that Allison may not argue, cry, or attack. In that case, simply repeat your words calmly, and gently end the conversation.

Another way to handle it is less courageous, but easier. You can simply be less and less available and let the friendship die a natural death. The important thing is that you realize that any friendship that makes you feel less than who you know you are and pulls you down is not worth cultivating or continuing. However, dealing with toxic relationships in family members is trickier. In the case of your mother-in-law, or any toxic family member, you could try a few strategies:

- Share your concerns. "Mom, it hurts my feelings when you make comments about my house." Your mother-in-law may be surprised (or feel guilty) that her comments have hurt you and she may turn over a new leaf. But don't count on it.

- If she doesn't turn over a new leaf, consider setting stronger boundaries. Let her know in firm but respectful terms that you will no longer listen to her comments.

- As a last resort and to protect yourself, limit your interactions with your mother-in-law to as few as necessary. Remember that you are protecting your wellbeing. And to do so means not subjecting yourself to toxic relationships. This does not mean that you limit the contact of your spouse or your children to your mother-in-law. It means that you limit your own contact to what feels comfortable for you. What this does is reclaim your life, and let your mother-in-law know that you understand what she is doing and that you have chosen not to accept it.

## A Diet of Young Nurses

Nurses eat their young. An interesting diet, considering that after nurses spit the latest novice nurse out of their mouth, they burp a bit and complain about the nursing shortage. I'm not sure why that is, other than misery loves company. Many older nurses figure, "Hey, I suffered when I started out; these new nurses should too."

Every generation of nurses has believed that the latest recruits are ill prepared and averse to working hard. And every group of new nurses has eventually proven their mettle and brought something better to the profession. We can't afford to lose enthusiastic and energetic novice nurses. And I think we all know that.

For the novice nurse who fears he can't make it through one more shift feeling like the lowest life form to slide across a linoleum floor – this too shall pass. But that probably doesn't soothe and salve the hurt and humiliation you feel every day.

First, let me welcome you to the nursing profession. You will never find another profession that offers you the versatility and creativity and the opportunity to make a difference in people's lives that nursing provides. But first we need to shore you up.

Make a list of the skills you bring to work everyday. Be specific, and don't stop until you've listed ten:

1.

2.

3.

4.

5.

6.

7.

8.

9.

10.

Now, write down what you hope to bring to patient care. Be as descriptive and concrete as possible. Why is that important to you?

_____

_____

_____

_____

_____

_____

Whenever you are feeling eaten up and spit out at work, review the list of skills and your statement about what you hope to bring to patient care. And add to your list of skills as it grows – and it will.

When you feel used and abused by an experienced nurse, try a nonconfrontational conversation with the offending nurse in language that recognizes the nurse as a valuable mentor and invites him or her to help you. You want to give him or her every opportunity to stop the intimidating behavior and get that nurse in your corner:

"Linda, I know I have so much to learn, and I hope that I can count on you to help me become as skilled a nurse as you. Do you have any suggestions that could help me accelerate my learning?"

Most novice nurses are afraid to confront their abuser. And that's what it is – abuse. But as you can see from the example above, a confrontation doesn't have to be an ugly scene. You can make it work for you.

Another strategy to consider is finding a mentor – a skilled and experienced nurse who would be willing to guide you through your practice and be your cheerleader.

If your workplace does not offer mentors, meet with your nurse manager and ask his recommendations of experienced nurses who might be willing to work with you. Seek out experienced nurses who can show you the ropes and guide you along the path.

Ask yourself, "Where am I lacking? What skills need beefing up? What steps could I take to enhance and improve my practice?" Join a professional nursing association and network. Read nursing magazines and journals to continue to improve and increase your knowledge base. Take classes offered by your workplace or nearby healthcare facilities. A diploma in hand does not a nurse make.

Finally, remember to mentor those who come after you. It's only fair. For the experienced nurse who subsists on a diet of novice nurses – you need to change your eating habits! Here's a strategy to try instead: Take a novice under your wing and mentor her into the nurse you want caring for you in your old age. Because one thing's for sure, you may not need a nurse caring for you now, but it's pretty certain you'll need one in the future.

## Building a Village

We've all heard that it takes a village to raise a child. It's a great sentiment in that it reminds us that we all have an individual and a collective responsibility to the world. In other words, we are not an island. We do not create, live, work, play, or love in a vacuum. We need other people.

Building a village or creating a community is an important part of our personal and professional success. Our personal community might be made up of friends or like-minded people. Our professional community might be made up of colleagues, professional association members, and mentors.

The power of community can change you. You might consider starting a group of nurse colleagues committed to supporting each other toward a successful nursing career. You could:

1. Ask permission to hold meetings in a room at your healthcare facility. The meeting could be held an hour before or after your shift on a regular basis.

2. Put up posters about the group.

3. Set up ground rules. For instance, only 5-10 minutes of whining or complaining.

4. Invite guest speakers to address the group on success strategies (president of a nursing association, expert on public speaking/writing, image consultant, or marketing expert).

Community is not just a career strategy. Having fun and pursuing interests is a great way to add a sense of balance to your life, especially when you work in a pressure-cooker career like nursing. If you're 50-years-or more and female, you might consider joining a local chapter of the Red Hat Society. This is an international club that has fun as its driving philosophy. All members are required to wear red hats (the more outlandish, the better) and purple outfits on all outings.

Having a sense of community can help us progress much more quickly because we have people behind us who support and encourage us to do more and be more than we think we're capable of becoming.

# Resources and Bibliography

Abaya, Carol. The Sandwich Generation©. Available at: http://www.thesandwichgeneration.com

Cardillo, Donna. *Your 1st Year As a Nurse*. Available through Donna Cardillo & Associates at: www.dcardillo.com.

Elder care. Available at: www.elderweb.com.

Internet Community of Elder Caregivers. Available at: www.ec-online.net

Meals on Wheels Association of America. Available at: www.mowaa.org

National Center on Women and Aging. Available at: www.brandeis.edu/heller/national/ind.html

National Institute on Aging. Available at: www.nih.gov/nia

National Adult Day Services Association. Available at: www.nadsa.org

Nursing organizations. See chapter Six.

Red Hat Society. Available at: www.redhatsociety.com.

Schloss, SD. *Taking Care of Mom, Taking Care of Me*. Judiaca Press. 2002.

# Chapter Three

# A Bolus of Self-Care

"I want to laugh. I want lightness in the world. I want it to be more fun."
Whoopi Goldberg

It's hard to turn around in any bookstore these days without knocking a self-help book off the shelves. Self-care is the buzzword of this decade, because technology has launched our world into hyper speed.

Self-care has shown up on our radar screens because there is now a realization that living life at warp speed does not a good life make. Technology, which was supposed to make our lives easier, has provided us with the ability to take on even more work. We work harder and faster, but with a lingering sense that something is missing. And what is missing is often ourselves.

It's difficult to live a truly fulfilled life without understanding what our needs are and how to best meet them. And the opposite is also true. If we take good care of ourselves, we have the time to reflect, consider, dream, and act on plans that can bring us fulfillment in our personal and professional lives.

Let's look at how we might better care for ourselves.

## The Downside of Humility

"Who me? Ah shucks, it's nothing. I'm just doing what nurses do." If those words have ever passed your lips, go to your room.

Seriously, humility has long been touted as a wonderful virtue we (usually defined as nurses, or women in general) should all strive for. Forget it! Humility has not done nurses or the nursing profession any great favors. If anything, humility has held the profession back by presenting nurses as subservient, task-oriented, order takers who do so with a smile on our face, and grateful for any nods passed our way.

When's the last time you met a humble surgeon? Humility in small doses can be charming, but in liberal doses it makes the person wearing the humble pie appear weak and ineffective. And who wants a weak and ineffective person for a healthcare provider? Most of us feel much more comfortable with a confidant and effective person championing our healthcare. Too much is at stake.

Nursing is an interesting profession. On one hand we want the world to view us as highly educated and skilled healthcare providers; on the other hand we drop our heads and refuse to acknowledge our education and skilled expertise. Ain't nothing, ma'am.

You can't have it both ways. You're either willing to acknowledge and claim your expertise and stride confidently onto the practice setting and the healthcare landscape, or you're going to have to raise the white flag, surrender, and admit that we're just order-taking, task-oriented servants of the healthcare system. If the second option doesn't appeal to you, then it's time to fish or cut bait. Our profession and your self-esteem as a healthcare professional are riding on it.

So, where do we begin? We begin with you. It all starts on the inside and works its way out and to the profession. You can't count on your colleagues doing this for you. Think like the US Army – their slogan is "An Army of One." The military understands that you can't have a powerful military without individual soldiers who see themselves as the best, the brightest, and the most prepared. It must first begin with the individual.

Still, many nurses hang onto their humility out of fear. What will people think of me? Who am I to take credit? People will think I'm full of myself. That may be true, but if it is true it's because those "other people" we worry about so much suffer from humility as well. You need to show them the way. Teach by example.

Let's take a look at your fears and get them out into the open. Be as descriptive as possible, and write down exactly what you fear will happen by letting your humility go. What's the worst that could happen?

_____

_____

_____

_____

_____

Now, imagine that you've cast your fears aside. You're no longer willing to be humble. When you do something well, you take credit for it. When someone compliments you, you accept it graciously and in a matter-of-fact manner. Describe in detail how you think that would feel. How do you suppose it would impact you and your professional career?

———————————————————
———————————————————
———————————————————
———————————————————

Do you feel a difference with the above two scenarios? Can you see how the second scenario would make a difference in who you think you are and how others perceive you? Now what's stopping you?

Take a moment and list the clinical skills you believe set you apart. Don't stop until you have listed at least twenty.

| | |
|---|---|
| 1. | 11. |
| 2. | 12. |
| 3. | 13. |
| 4. | 14. |
| 5. | 15. |
| 6. | 16. |
| 7. | 17. |
| 8. | 18. |
| 9. | 19. |
| 10. | 20. |

Now, list the professional skills you possess that you think represent the best of professional nurses. Don't stop until you've listed ten.

1.
2.
3.
4.
5.
6.
7.
8.
9.
10.

The reason I wanted you to list the above clinical and professional skills is because it's important to understand your skill level and to reassess where you stand on a regular basis. And it's a boost for your self-esteem to see, in black and white, what makes you such a good, professional nurse. If you write it down, there is no denying it; it's right there in front of your eyes.

How many times has a patient complimented you on some extraordinary thing you did, or a colleague patted you on the back for making a good call or averting a disastrous patient outcome? Chances are it has happened and you've waved it away as if it didn't count. That must stop today. Right now.

Nursing is one of the best-kept secrets in healthcare. And it's probably true for two reasons – 1) nurses have perpetuated the self-sacrificing caregiver role, and 2) in some respects, the healthcare system prefers that nurses remain that way because it makes it easier to control them and not recognize them as the true stars of healthcare. Ask yourself, Don't you get just a wee bit tired of the media's love affair with physicians? Don't you think that if the media understood what nurses really do, perhaps nurses and nursing might be portrayed more realistically as the heroes of healthcare that they are?

Get ready to change it now. One nurse at a time. Here are some ways to begin:

1.  Make sure that your personnel file represents all that you've accomplished and achieved. If you've published, presented, planned and executed some program, or received great feedback from a patient – make sure it is in your file (and that you've got your own file going at home with duplicates of everything).

2.  The next time you are complimented by a patient, look the patient in the eyes, smile, and say 'thank you.' Tell the patient that experiences like this happen all the time. And that it is not to say that the patient's experience is not extraordinary, but that nurses do extraordinary things every day, many times a day – and that you appreciate it that he or she noticed.

3.  If you did something well, claim it. It doesn't mean you are bragging. You're just stating a fact. And to be fair, make sure you create an environment where your colleagues feel comfortable doing the same. If you noticed a colleague doing a great job, comment on it and don't allow him or her to be humble.

4.  Educate your public relations department about the great things you and your nurse colleagues do. Get together with your nurse colleagues

and nurse manager and invite the PR person to coffee to educate him on the nursing role and encourage him to champion nursing in the community and within the facility. It's good business sense for a facility to tout the expertise of their staff to the community, and it provides an opportunity to spread the word about nursing. If nursing doesn't have a prominent place on your facility website, ask why not. Make sure that PR person understands what a powerful recruitment tool it is to have a strong nursing presence on the website, and the confidence it can inspire in healthcare consumers who are researching facilities that can best meet their needs.

5. If there is a facility newsletter, make sure that you are submitting accomplishments for publication. If an opportunity doesn't already exist, encourage your facility (talk to your nursing administrators and PR department) to include exemplars in the community newsletters. Explain that it is an opportunity to educate the community about the impact of quality nursing care. Encourage the facility to spotlight nurses in different practice areas in the newsletter and on the facility website.

Think back on your career in nursing. Has your humility improved patient care? Has it propelled your career forward in the way you expected? Do the people in your life look up to you as a skilled and knowledgeable professional deserving of respect and admiration?

If it's not working for you, it's time to take action.

## What Do You Need to Finish?

We all have things in our life that are unfinished. It might be the telemetry course or advanced degree you started and never finished, or the hallway closet that you never get around to cleaning out. It may be the unfinished conversation with someone who hurt you, or that idea you have for improving patient care that you've been meaning to write up and present. Some of the unfinished things that trap you in a quagmire of indecision and inaction may include things you've planned on getting around to, pounds you've meant to take off, conversations left unfinished, or relationships neglected or ended, and taking those necessary steps to move forward in your career.

When we have things in our life that remain unfinished we never are truly free in our own life. Unfinished and unresolved matters follow us wherever we go, attached to our psyche and hanging precariously above our head as an unpleasant reminder that we really don't have our act together. Sound familiar? Good, recognizing the problem is step one in correcting the situation once and for all.

The truth is, when you are finally able to finish those things that you're dragging endlessly around, you experience a lightness, a burst of energy, and certainly improved confidence. Your energy is freed up from dealing with the unresolved matters and is now a reserve ready to use for things you want to add to or enhance in your life. It's also true that being freed up from unfinished business gives you more time in your life and more opportunities, because the universe, in all its wisdom, understands that you are finally ready for more. If that sounds too woo-woo-this-is-way-too-far-out, consider this: the physical reality of having less hanging over your head and more time allows you to recognize an opportunity when it appears. Think about it. If your mind is clouded by thoughts of how you never finish anything – if I'd finished that telemetry course I could have transferred to CCU by now – how likely would it be for you to notice the small classified ad for an internship in CCU? Probably slim. And, if you did see it, your critical mind would remind you of how you failed the last time you tried to move toward your dream career goal.

Why not create a different reality for yourself? Now is probably a good time to bring up unfinished matters in your life, such as traumas or inappropriate actions you took or judgments you made, addictions, and so forth. These are situations that need to be handled and dealt with once and for all – but not in this book. These serious matters may be holding you back, but to find your way beyond them you need professional help from a psychiatric clinical nurse specialist or some other psychiatric healthcare provider. Navigating through such unfinished matters on your own, or with this book, will not resolve the issues that need to be addressed in a way that most meets your needs. So, get that taken care of now.

How do you finish what is unfinished? Step by step. By putting one foot in front of the other; one small action followed by another small action. Let's say you never finished that telemetry course. You've practiced in med/surg for years and really have always wanted to practice in the CCU. But laziness, lack of time, and a host of other reasons you can't recall caused you to drop out of the course. It's haunted you ever since. You think about the wasted money, the wasted time, and the drop in your confidence level. Maybe it's just not meant to be, you tell yourself.

29

Lets finish this. First, tell yourself, you "failed" to complete the course, but that was then and this is now. You're older, wiser, and certainly smarter. Tell yourself that you're going to create a new reality – that you can finish that course and you can prepare yourself to move to CCU.

Second, list all the possible ways you can prepare yourself for moving into the CCU. Research your facility – do they have internships in the CCU? Do they offer continuing education courses for the critical care units? What about courses at local colleges or universities that could prepare you? Perhaps you could contact the Association of Critical Care Nurses <www.aacn.org> for more information. Or perhaps you could ask to speak to the CCU manager and ask her advice for preparing yourself for working in the unit. Whom else could you talk to for information?

Third, look at your list. What can you do today that will bring you one step closer to your dream job? Do it, and then move on to the next step. Does this guarantee that you will get a job in CCU? Of course not. But what it does guarantee is that you have finished what needed to be finished and you have moved closer to your goal of making it happen. You've chosen to take charge of the situation rather than letting the situation continue to take charge of you.

Okay, let's take something a bit stickier – relationships, for instance. Let's say that you made some unkind remarks about one of your nurse colleagues, and she heard about it. Since then your relationship has been strained and uncomfortable for both of you, and you regret your words and the situation. What could you do to finish or resolve this?

First, for yourself – accept responsibility. Recognize the full consequences of your actions or words and how that diminished you in your own eyes. Recognize that the actions and words of before do not fully represent who you are today or who you want to be. It's important that you are honest with yourself so you don't create the same unfinished situation in the future. Even if you rationalized at the time that the other person deserved your words or actions, it's important to recognize that you are responsible and accountable for your part in this.

Next, speak to that person, either in person or on the phone, and accept responsibility for your actions or words.

"Janet, I said something hurtful about you that I regret and it has created an uncomfortable situation between us. I want you to know that I am deeply sorry and I want to make it right between us again."

Janet may forgive and forget and you can both move on. Or she may hold a grudge. That is her choice. You only own your behavior, not hers. But what you've done is finish an unresolved matter for yourself, accepted culpability, and cleared the air. You are free to move on.

Your turn. Name an unfinished matter you have not resolved.

_____

_____

_____

_____

That was then, this is now. List all the ways you can think of that would help finish your unresolved matter. You don't have to do all these things, just brainstorm a list.

_____

_____

_____

_____

_____

Take a look at your list. What one step on your list could you take today that would bring you closer to finishing this matter? Or what conversation could you have that would clear the air? Write it down. Next to it, write down the date you'll complete each step by.

_____

_____

_____

_____

Great. Now take that step. If that one step doesn't "finish" it, go back and pick another step and take action. Continue until you have resolved the matter in your mind and you consider it a done deal. Congratulations!

**Build Reserves – Time, Money, Energy, Opportunities**

Nurses are probably the hardest-working providers in healthcare. The pace is unrelenting and daunting. The patient care is nonstop and exhausting. The expectations and stress seem to grow each day. And that's just your work environment! At home, your responsibilities continue and your reserve of energy, time, and money is stretched to the limit. It doesn't have to be that way.

When you feel stretched to the max, it's hard to imagine that there could be an easier way to do things; a less stressful existence. It's always been that way, and it's getting worse. How can you expect anything different? The idea is to move from a place of scarcity – that's how it's always been and it's only going to get worse – to a place of reserve – I have everything I need and I am the author of my life.

It's interesting, but some people I talk to are uncomfortable with the idea of their lives being anything but chaotic. They don't believe that they deserve anything easy. You may know people like this. They live with one crisis after another. They become a magnetic force that pulls to them every crisis you can imagine. You wonder, How do they live on sheer adrenaline like that?

Are they a lost cause? No. For them, it can be helpful if they change their belief system and "fake it until they make it," by telling themselves that they deserve to live a less chaotic life and then act as if that is the case. And then by taking action toward that belief system, they essentially make it so.

Here's a simple example of faking it until you make it. Samantha is an ED staff nurse who has an interest in helmet safety. As a result of her interest and her nurse manager's prodding, she has been asked to share her expertise at a community safety meeting. Her anxiety level is sky high and she is dreading it. She doesn't doubt her knowledge base, only her ability to stand center stage and speak to such a large group. How can she fake it until she makes it?

Here are the steps:

1.  Prepare her presentation so that she knows what to say, and how she's going to say it. She can decide on what tools will help her feel more comfortable. For instance, will using a Power Point presentation make it easier for her or is she more comfortable with a lower-tech method, such as index cards or a prepared speech?

2.  Rehearse until she feels she knows the presentation.

3.  Develop a mantra (in the present tense, as it if it is already true) – "I am a competent speaker and the audience is enjoying and learning." Also, Samantha can practice visualizing herself walking confidently on to the stage, delivering her presentation, and hearing the audience clapping enthusiastically.

4.  When it's time for the presentation, Samantha can repeat her mantra to herself and then "act as if it is true" when she takes the stage. Is it possible that she'll make a mistake? Yes. But, it's far more likely that by preparing, visualizing, and telling herself that she is a competent speaker, she will succeed beyond her expectations and discover something about herself in the process.

Time is finite. You can't make more time in your day. But what you can do is rearrange your time, manipulate it so that it makes more sense for you. Time is a strange thing. Though each minute is exactly 60 seconds, how you interpret time or that minute can be quite different. If you're in pain, for example, a minute can seem excruciatingly long. However, if you've just won all the free merchandise you can throw in a shopping cart in a minute; that minute is going to seem far shorter than 60 seconds. How you interpret and think about time influences whether you believe you have abundance or a shortage.

Let's look at some strategies for creating a reserve of time in your life. First we have to figure out where we are losing or wasting time.

On a separate piece of paper, map out your day. What's a typical day look like? Write down your schedule with a rough estimate of the time and be specific about what you are doing.

5:00 AM: Walk the dog, shower, breakfast.
6:30 AM: Get kids ready for school bus.
Continue until you've itemized a typical day.

The idea is that by really defining how you spend your time from rising in the morning until bedtime, you can see exactly what is eating up your day, and you can see where in the day or evening you are not using time to your best advantage. This is where you can make a decision to manipulate your time. Some ideas for manipulating time based on the above example:

1.  Set out your clothes the night before. Have your children set out their clothes, too.

2.  If you pack a lunch to work, make that the night before.

3. Take turns with a neighbor to make sure her kids and your kids get the school bus in the morning. That will give you a couple of mornings a week with a window of "free" time.

4. Have your children take turns cleaning up the kitchen after breakfast, or doing a quick straighten up before you're all out the door.

Other ideas for manipulating time:

1. Get a housekeeper to do the heavy cleaning once every two weeks. If that's out of your budget, consider swapping cleaning chores with a friend. She cleans your house twice a month and you have the month 'off.' The next month you clean her house twice. Or turn it into an opportunity to socialize and help each other clean. You can talk and clean in half the time. You might even enlist a group of friends or neighbors to do this.

2. Start a babysitting cooperative. Get a group of friends or neighbors with kids, and take turns watching the kids. All the moms will have some free time without kids to spend as they wish.

3. Shop in bulk. Set one day or evening aside to buy a reserve of items you frequently need to make shopping runs for: toilet paper, paper towels, cleaning supplies, contact lens solution, greeting cards (birthday, anniversary, get well, sympathy, congratulations, and blank cards), stamps, laundry detergent, nylon stockings, food items you can freeze until you need it (i.e., bread), shampoo and condition, toothpaste, and so forth. Organize a place to keep your reserves and you'll waste less time running to the grocery store. If you get a reserve of food, especially nonperishable items, you'll spend less time with your regular grocery shopping.

4. Make appointments well in advance. When you have a physical, make your next appointment before you leave the office. Make a succession of hair appointments, rather than trying to fit an appointment in at the last minute or finding that your favorite hairdresser is taking a vacation and your roots are showing.

5.   Avoid wasting time trying to manage clutter and chaos. Maintain your house (remember to enlist the cooperation of your spouse and children). Make it a family rule that everyone makes a sweep of the house before going to bed – put away toys, straighten kitchen, empty dishwasher, toss newspapers, and so forth. In the morning, same thing. Keep bathrooms neat and clean between heavy duty cleaning, take a few minutes to swish the toilet with the toilet bowl brush (keep half mixture of cleaning solution and water in the toilet bowl brush holder), and then use a disposable cleaning cloth to wipe down the sink and then the toilet. Straighten the towels and empty the wastebasket. The bathrooms will always smell nice and stay clean between heavy cleaning.

6.   Use your time to and from work. Listen to classical music to de-stress. "Read" that book you've been meaning to get to – use books on tape to listen to in the car. Books on tape are available to buy, rent, or borrow from your local library. You'll find you won't mind the traffic to or from work. You can also use tapes or CDs to learn a new language, listen to motivational speakers, or study for that exam (read your notes into a tape and then play it while you drive).

7.   Periodically – at least twice a year – de-clutter closets. Be ruthless in your clothes closet. If it doesn't fit, if you haven't worn it in a year, if the color doesn't suit you, if you don't absolutely love it – throw it out or donate it to someone who can use it. Most people tend to keep their closets packed to the gills with clothing that no longer meets their needs. It's a waste of time and a waste of money. There are people who could get a lot of use out of those clothes. Keep your clothes streamlined, clean, and in good repair. Buy only colors that suit you and clothing that fits and flatters you. If you keep key elements in your closet that suit your lifestyle, you'll always have what you need when you need it.

8.   Get rid of your laundry. If you have children older than 12, they can do their own laundry – and maybe even your laundry. Make the rule in your house – launder, fold, and put away.

9.   Assign a designated cook. When children reach a certain age, let them take turns cooking one night a week. Once they get use to it, they'll find they like using their imagination to come up with adventuresome

meals, and you get to sit for a while with your feet up and smell a delicious meal wafting from the kitchen.

10. Avoid vegging out in front of the television at night. You may feel you've earned it, but it may not be the best way to manipulate your time. Be discriminating about what television you want to watch. Then think of the rest of your television-watching time as money – and spend it the way you want to. You could read, call a friend, meet your sister at the local coffee shop, go to a bookstore, attend a poetry slam, call your mother, balance your checkbook, give yourself a facial, or just sit alone and think!

## A Reserve of Money

Many people have an interesting and adversarial relationship with money. They live with the belief that money is scarce and will most likely always be scarce. That's just the way it is, they think, and it's not going to change. Many people also try to make themselves feel better about not having as much money as they'd like by demonizing money and people who have money.

"Aw, she's probably so busy with her money that she doesn't care about anyone or anything."
"At least I'm happy the way I am. That man is probably miserable."
"Money makes people do strange things. You're just better off without it."

The truth is, money doesn't corrupt, cause people to neglect their loved ones, or make people miserably unhappy. People do that. Money is an inanimate object. What is true is that your beliefs about money are far more powerful than the money itself. And if your belief is that money corrupts or causes you to suddenly be miserable, there is little likelihood that you are going to take any actions that would bring more money into your life. Why would you want to be more miserable? Instead, you constantly make that belief right by sabotaging yourself on a subconscious level of awareness. Unlike what many people believe, money is not the root of all evil. The love of money is the root of all evil. Money is simply a form of currency or a tool to get our needs, and hopefully our wants, met.

It is certainly beyond the scope of this book to offer financial advice, but what I can do is get you to question your beliefs about money and set the wheels in motion to get more money into your life and make it work for you – not the other way around.

So let's see what your belief is about money. Perhaps it's something you've never taken the time to think about, but it's a necessary step to bringing more money into your life.

List all the beliefs you have about money and what money represents to you. Were there any beliefs about money that you heard while growing up? What did money mean to your family? Be specific.

Money means:

_____
_____
_____
_____
_____
_____
_____

Now, when you look at the beliefs you have listed above. What is the one overriding belief that you hold?

_____


Is your belief about money a belief that you think has served you well? Has it helped to bring all the money you need into your life? Or is it possible that your belief has sabotaged you in some way?

If your belief has sabotaged you it is also possible to develop a new belief about money that will make you more receptive to receiving it into your life. All you have to do is believe the opposite of your long-held belief. If, for instance, you believed that money is the root of all evil, you need to select a belief that is more positive. An example might be, "Money brings me unlimited opportunities to make my life better." Or, "Money allows me to give to myself and others."

Write down your new belief about money. Remember that writing it down is not enough. You must exchange your old belief about money with this new one. Let it become a mantra for you.

My new belief about money:

_____

Write your new belief on slips of paper and put it in your wallet, where you keep your bills, and in your checkbook to remind you and put you into a positive frame of mind.

Now that you have developed a new relationship with money, it's time to tackle the nitty-gritty of creating a reserve of money in your life. A mantra will help, but you have to be an active member in this new relationship with money. There are a number of resources at the end of this chapter to help you continue to develop this relationship and create your monetary reserve.

To make money, you have to save money. No groaning. The fact is that to create a reserve of money you must understand its value. If you understand its value, you will also understand that it is disrespectful to waste money and treat it callously. The first step is to look at the ways in your life that you can save money. Saving money is creating a reserve.

Here are some tips. The resources at the end of this chapter will discuss these tips in more detail:

1. Create a budget.
2. Use coupons when grocery shopping.
3. Wait for sales before making a purchase.
4. Take your lunch to work instead of buying it.
5. Make your own coffee instead of stopping at the gourmet coffee shop.
6. Save all the change in your wallet. You'll be surprised how quickly it adds up.
7. Eat out less often.
8. Rent a movie instead of going to the movie theater.
9. Buy the best you can afford. Buying cheap usually ends up needing to be replaced.
10. Instead of going out to dinner with friends, invite them to dinner at your house.
11. Leave charge cards at home when shopping. Avoid impulse buying.
12. Have at least 10% of your paycheck automatically deducted to save in a retirement or savings plan.
13. Never buy anything unless you absolutely love it or unless it absolutely adds to the quality of your life.
14. Barter for things. If you are an awesome cook, consider bartering your expertise with your neighbor who can make those custom curtains you want. Or

offer to babysit for a weekend in exchange for your friend, the electrician, putting up your new light.
15. Pay down your charge cards – to $0!

Saving money is all about respecting money and what it means. If you don't learn to respect it, money has an uncanny way of slipping out of your wallet and through your fingers. Money is currency earned through your blood, sweat, and tears in the workplace. Disrespecting that money is disrespecting the hard work you put into earning that it. You are well aware of how hard you work to earn your paycheck. You should be just as aware and respectful of how that money is spent. When money is disrespected, it is spent easily and without thought of the consequences. One important thing to keep in mind – by improving our relationship with money, we also provide good modeling to the children in our life so that they, too, can develop a positive and respectful understanding of its value.

To develop strategies for making money, it is always wise to seek professional counsel, such as a financial expert or financial planner. Often times, the most dire situation can be turned around with professional help. One example of this is Susan.

Susan is an ED nurse who works part-time evenings. Her husband was downsized from his engineering job. Two months, six months, a year went by with no new job prospects. Susan took on as many hours as she could, but their bills and high charge debt increased while their savings dwindled to nothing. And then the unimaginable happened – they lost their home and had to declare bankruptcy. Susan and her husband were depressed and defeated. They had three kids and no home. They moved in with relatives until Susan's husband found a new job and they were more financially stable. Determined to buy a home and build their life again, they sat down with a financial planner. For the first time in their married lives, they worked as a team, sacrificing where they could and following the planner's goals to the letter. Susan sold her car and bought a cheaper, second-hand car. They started accounts and faithfully put money into each account – car account, savings account, miscellaneous house upkeep account, vacation account, weekly allowance account, and so forth. If the money wasn't in a specific account, they didn't buy it.

Today, Susan and her husband have a lovely home. They remodeled a playroom – and paid cash. They take vacations – and pay cash. Susan still drives a second-hand car and won't replace it until enough money is in her car account so she can pay cash for the car.

By respecting the money they earned, saving where they could, and buying items mindful of the transaction between hard labor and a product, they now have a modest reserve of money. They understand how easy it is to buy now, pay later – and how easily that can come back to haunt you.

## A Reserve of Energy

Creating a reserve of energy is closely tied up with manipulating time and having a reserve of money. A lack of either of those things can weigh us down and stress us out, which causes a natural depletion of energy. Assuming that your time manipulation is in order and your reserve of money is healthy, we can move on to creating a reserve of energy.

To create a reserve of energy, it's important to do a health risk assessment. Any number of acute and chronic conditions can deplete your natural reserves of energy. So it goes without saying that regular physical assessments are critical to the equation. If you have unmanaged health problems or lack regular health assessments, that must be your first order of business. Tend to what needs tending; fix what needs fixing.

Obvious physical things that affect energy levels that need to be addressed:

1. Overweight
2. Alcohol or other drug problems
3. Mental disorders (i.e., depression)
4. Dysfunctional relationships
5. Lack of exercise

If one or more of the above listed physical things rise to the top of your list, you will need to tackle them right away. Obviously, you may need professional help for any or all of those items. But there is no question that every one of them contributes to sucking the energy right out of your life. They drag you down and make it difficult to work and live fully and with vigor. As nurses, you are well aware of the resources available to you to deal with these issues. And often those resources are right under your nose – where you work!

Let's consider one of the above serious energy drains. Remember that this list often requires professional help. But let's simplify it for a moment so that you can see the larger picture.

Thomas is an OR nurse. He's 25 pounds overweight, has back problems, and most days when he gets home he just crashes on his couch. Thomas feels depleted by his workday. Standing on his feet for long hours has taken its toll. He feels guilty about his lack of energy; he would much rather play catch with his children and help his wife out with dinner. But his lack of energy seems to win each day as he consumes a bag of potato chips and slumps on the sofa surfing the television channels. What strategies might Thomas put into play?

- Get a physical to rule out any physical causes for his weight and lethargy. Also, get clearance from the nurse practitioner to begin a sensible exercise program.

- Eat a sensible, balanced diet. Instead of the bag of potato chips, try fresh vegetables and dip. Keep vegetables clean, chopped and ready to eat.

- Avoid food temptations. Pack a lunch and healthy snacks, or buy a healthy salad in the cafeteria.

- Take a 20-minute walk before driving home. This will decrease the stress from the workday, establish a workout plan, and make sure that Thomas arrives home ready to play with his children and help his wife in the kitchen. To make sure that his wife has the same opportunities, Thomas could help the children with their homework while his wife exercises for 20 minutes. When the children are old enough to be alone in the house, Thomas and his wife can take a walk together and get an opportunity to connect at the end of the day – and get in shape at the same time!

- Begin a weight-training program. Thomas could get advice from an expert (i.e., physical trainer) on how best to strengthen his muscles – in particular his abdominal muscles, legs, and back.

Often, when we suffer from an energy drain, it's difficult to see the solution because our chronic fatigue makes it difficult to see beyond the most obvious – our lack of energy. But there is often a solution, and it is sometimes as simple as focusing our attention to our life and making a plan of action.

There are often small energy drains in our life that sap away at our vigor a little at a time. Clutter is one of them. We live in a society of conspicuous consumption. Magazines, newspapers, television, and radio are constantly hyping the next best thing we absolutely must have. Just walk through the grocery store and you'll see aisles and aisles of choices that citizens in most other countries can only dream about. And while we're busy consuming and acquiring, we are also busy working. Magazines we've been meaning to read pile up, closets become cramped with clothes we don't have time to wear – or don't even like anymore. Bathroom drawers become cramped with outdated makeup and containers filled with potions we've forgotten about. The family room is filled with toys that have long been outgrown and gadgets with batteries that died two years ago. Clutter fills every room and weighs us down as we mentally remind ourselves that we really need to get to that someday and clean out the rubble.

That clutter psychologically drains our energy every time we look at it and every time we try our darndest not to look at it. It reminds us that we really don't have things under control after all.

The good news is that a clutter problem is a pretty simple thing to fix, and the rewards are immediate. And most of us would be better served by addressing any clutter in our lives. It creates space – physical and psychological – in our homes and in our heads.

Some de-clutter tips:

- Bedroom closets. If you haven't worn it in a year – throw it away or give it away. If it doesn't flatter you – ditto.

- Bathroom closets. Discard all out-dated medications, make-up, and toiletries. Wipe down all drawers and organize all items. Ask yourself, Do I really need five different bottles of opened shampoos?

- Toss out out-dated magazines and newspapers. If there's an interesting article or recipe you want to save, just tear it out and file it. With the Internet, we seldom need to save magazines, newspapers, and catalogs anymore.

- Clean out your car. If it's a landfill on wheels and you feel embarrassed offering anyone a ride – clean it out.

- Clean off kitchen counters. Give yourself room to create.

- Explore the deep recesses of your refrigerator and clean it out.

- Weed out toys. If it's not used, stop stepping over it and donate it to someone who can use it.

- Don't handle paperwork more than once. When your mail comes, open it and make a decision – handle, file, or discard.

All of the above strategies are simple to do, and the temptation is to think Hmmm…what's the big deal? How can cleaning out my car give me more energy? The difference is in how it makes us feel. Here's an example: A colleague asks you for a ride home after work. You say yes, of course, but your mind immediately pictures your car littered with empty fast food containers, the drycleaning you've been meaning to drop off, muddy soccer shoes, and enough dog hair to knit a blanket. You know your colleague is grateful for the ride home, but oh, how you wish you had gotten around to cleaning out the car. That's a psychic drain. And easily remedied. For example, make it a rule that no one in your family leaves belongings in the car. As family members exit the car, they carry and put away their stuff.

What's draining you? List three things that are draining you and the strategies you can put into place to address them:

#1 drain_____

Strategy:
_____
_____
_____

#2 drain _____

Strategy:
_____
_____
_____

#3 drain _____

Strategy:

_____
_____
_____

When you've solved the first three energy drains, feel free to move on to any other drains.

## A Reserve of Opportunities

Someone once said, "The only place you can find success before work is in the dictionary." With that said, creating a reserve of opportunities is seldom the result of luck and more often the result of focused attention or hard work. The good news is that we can be the creators of opportunities and that often it is just being open to receiving or accepting an opportunity.

How many opportunities have you missed in your life because you weren't ready or were asleep at the wheel of your life and didn't even recognize the opportunity when it was in front of you?

People who seem to have more opportunities than we do, who seem luckier than we are, are usually people who pay attention to their world and to the possibilities around them. And they are usually people who seem to "make things happen" by creating opportunities. No one would ever accuse them of being asleep at the wheel. Rather, they are acutely aware of every twist in the road, shortcut, and direct route to their goals. They understand that opportunities are really action steps in motion!

Liz has worked on a med/surg floor for the past year. She ultimately wants to become a psychiatric clinical nurse specialist.

Sonya has worked in the OR for the past six months. She ultimately wants to become a forensics nurse.

Fast-forward five years. Liz is a psychiatric clinical nurse specialist and enjoys working with her clients. Sonya is still working in the OR and dreads going to work every day. She's thinking about leaving the nursing profession.

What happened? How did Liz acquire her dream and Sonya miss out? Sonya says that she has rotten luck. No opportunities appeared before her, and she doesn't understand how Liz got so lucky. Sonya was always meaning to research colleges that have forensic programs for nurses, but she was too busy.

Here's what Liz did:

- Shared her dream with other nurses so that more eyes were scouting for opportunities to move her toward her goal.

- Understood that a strong med/surg background would be invaluable in the psychiatric setting. Met with her med/surg nurse manager and shared her ultimate goal and that she would like opportunities to improve her med/surg skills and psyche assessment skills.

- Met with a psychiatric clinical nurse specialist and did an informational interview. Liz asked the CNS the following: What skills would best serve Liz's goals? What educational preparation did he recommend? What did he like most and least about his career choice? What next steps would he recommend to Liz to help her move forward with her goal?

- Selected a psychiatric CNS mentor willing to work with her toward her goal.

- Followed through with the information she gathered and took action.

Two nurses, two goals. Yet only Liz was "lucky" enough to reach her goal. Liz had a reserve of opportunities because she didn't wait for them to magically appear. She created them. We all know people like Sonya, who blame the universe for their lack of opportunities. Remember that opportunities are action steps in motion, whether we create those action steps, as Liz did, or are open and willing to take action when an opportunity presents itself.

What career opportunity would you like to see before you?

_____

How could you make this career opportunity happen? What steps could you take that would bring you closer to this goal?

_____
_____
_____
_____
_____
_____
_____

Take a look at your strategies for making your goal happen. Take it one step further and ask yourself, When could I complete this step? By giving yourself a timetable for achieving each step, you are putting into play a real plan to create your opportunity.

Step one: _____
By when? _____

Step two: _____
By when? _____

Step three: _____
By when?_____

Creating opportunities is putting the work before success. It is also all about having a commitment to your future and a belief in yourself. Developing a strategy is not enough. You also have to make it real and set a time limit on it. And when you do that, opportunities will just happen to appear. It's not magic. It's creating that forward momentum that will propel you towards your dream.

**The Power of Beauty**

Beauty is not a word that usually springs to mind when thinking of nursing and patient care. But that doesn't mean it's not important. Beauty has a great healing property. It soothes the eyes of the beholder, inspires creative talent to strive for genius, and generally creates a feeling of relaxation and well being. Beauty has sent armies into battle and caused people to weep in appreciation.

Have you ever seen a painting that so moved you that you wept? Or saw flowers growing by the roadside, so brilliant and beautiful?

Yet we seldom see beauty around us in the patient care setting. Rather we see the ugliness in illness and injury. But there is a lot of beauty in your practice, hidden behind the stress and strain of too much to do in too little time.

There is beauty in the toothless smile of a grateful 92-year-old patient, the birth of a healthy baby, and in a peaceful and accepting death. Beauty is all around us. Sometimes we have to look for it – hard. Other times it hits us between the eyes. Beauty is such an important element in living a fulfilled personal and professional life. It is not a frivolous thing; it is necessary in our lives.

It's so important to have beauty in our homes. Our homes should be our respite, our safe harbor from the craziness in the world. After such a stressful day at work, you deserve to cross your front threshold and feel the rest of the world slip away. You don't need mountains of money to bring beauty into your home. Many times you don't need to spend a cent. Here are some tips to bring beauty into your life at home:

- Keep fresh flowers in your home where you can see and enjoy them. Don't use plastic flowers or plants. You need the energy from living flowers. Flowers can be expensive, so plant them and pick them from your garden. Or buy a single flower and put it in a little vase.

- De-clutter your home. Experiment with rearranging your furniture.

- Don't keep anything in your home, and don't buy anything, that you don't absolutely love. Your furniture and accessories should speak to you, should make you feel good.

- Use color. Pick colors that make you happy and paint an accent wall or a whole room.

- Enjoy nature around you. Take time in the morning to watch a sunrise. Or watch the sun set in the evening. Put a bird feeder near a window where you can see it.

- Play music that sets the mood you want in your home. Perhaps it's classical or jazz.

- Use scented candles to give your house a nice, inviting smell. Some people find the aroma of vanilla candles comforting. Remember to blow out candles when you are not in the room.

- Clean your windows frequently and let the sun come in.

You can have beauty in your home even if the home is small and your budget even smaller. One nurse I know has a tiny home, yet she created a beautiful oasis that looks like it cost much more than it did. She decided to limit her colors to two – white and blue – to give her small place a larger feel. Then she bought only what she could afford in those colors and only if she absolutely loved it. Bedside tables, beds, and coffee tables were salvaged from thrift shops and her local dump! She cleaned the furniture and painted them white, creating pieces that coordinate with each other. Every room is a blend of white furniture and blue fabrics of flowers and stripes. Accessories are either blue or white with touches of yellow here and there. All of it blends and flows together. The feel is airy and beautiful.

That sounds do-able, but you wonder how you can bring beauty into the workplace.

- Put a colorful flower where you can see it – your desk if you sit at one, or at the nurses' station.

- If permissible, play beautiful music softly in the background – i.e., classical.

- When at the nurses' station, keep your tea in a pretty mug rather than a Styrofoam cup. And keep aromatic herbal tea bags at work.

- Hang a beautiful picture at the nurses' station where you and everyone else can enjoy it. Oprah's magazine, *O Magazine*, has a stunning nature scene in every issue to inspire readers and encourage them to take a moment and breathe. When you're feeling particularly stressed, take a moment and lose yourself in the picture.

- If you have the luxury of a few moments to yourself. Step outside and breathe fresh air. Look for beauty.

- Encourage family members of patients to bring in bits of beauty to their loved ones' rooms. It doesn't have to be expensive roses. They can bring in a single brilliant Gerbera daisy or a few black-eyed Susans. There is something "happy" about those brilliantly colored flowers. Encourage the family to bring in a beautiful picture of nature – even torn from the pages of a magazine.

And don't neglect yourself in your search for beauty. It has nothing to do with vanity – or at least it shouldn't. It has to do with appreciating what you have and what you've been given. Pick colors that flatter you and make you feel good every time you put them on. Pick clothing styles that make you feel comfortable and attractive; clothing styles that you wear and that don't wear you. Think enough about yourself to keep yourself maintained and in good shape – just like you do your car.

Beauty adds so much to our lives, but sometimes we take it for granted or consider it unnecessary or frivolous. It is neither. Appreciating beauty and making an effort to bring beauty into your home and workplace is a way to add to the quality of your life. It's a way to stop the chaotic madness of life and pause to notice what is there. It's there, if we'll just take the time to look.

## Be Unreasonable

Nurses, on the whole, are a darn nice group of people. And what a mistake that has been!

Nurses have a reputation for being caring, self-sacrificing, nurturing, nice, reliable, hardworking, and honest. All positive attributes. Or are they? Words that don't come to mind when the public thinks of nurses are: autonomous, intelligent, lifesavers, educated, and strong.

The truth is that nurses are all of those things, and more. And there is one trait or characteristic usually attributed to nurses that has held the profession back and prevented the public from seeing all the attributes of nursing – niceness. Being nice has not served nursing, and nurses, well. Instead, what it has done is put down nursing, because in our culture niceness is seen as weak and inconsequential. And you know there is nothing inconsequential about nursing practice.

Nurses are the largest group of healthcare providers and the most invisible. In the eyes of the public, nurses are wonderful, order-taking robots. In the eyes of the media, nurses are second-class citizens of the healthcare industry. You know the drill...a nurse is a nurse is a nurse.... A nurse is an interchangeable unit that can be moved from one area of practice to the other. The practice is so undervalued by the public and some institutions that there is no understanding or appreciation for the body of knowledge in each area of practice. Who in their right mind would interchange physicians in the same way? Can you imagine someone with a cardiovascular problem going to see a dermatologist? It wouldn't happen because the public understands that physicians have expertise in certain areas of practice.

Being nice causes us to hold our tongues, accept what is unacceptable, and just bear what is because that's just what nurses do. Consider what would happen to the profession if nurses were unreasonable. By that I mean, strong and willing to go to the mat for themselves. Nurses have been known to stand up, but usually it's for their patients, seldom for themselves. Here's a new way to look at being unreasonable – strong boundaries; understanding of their own value (to the practice expertise and the bottom line); strong advocate for the patient and the profession of nursing; clear voice; clear vision and mission.

The problem with being considered nice is that it puts added pressure on you to continue to fulfill that expectation. How can you complain, disagree, put forth your own thoughts? People won't consider you as nice? It can't be done. The thing about being nice is that it's an externally determined attribute. Think about it. You can't call yourself nice, other people determine if you are nice or not. And usually, people consider you nice if you are meeting their needs. If you choose to meet your own needs, albeit politely, suddenly you find that you're no longer considered nice – you're considered selfish. In other words, you can't win if you're nice. Ever heard the old cliché – nice guys finish last? The fact is, they deserve to!

Think about the men and women you admire – Martin Luther King, Florence Nightingale, Mother Theresa, Oprah, and so forth. These people did not achieve greatness by being nice. Had they been nice people, they would never dare to follow their paths to greatness, because it would have meant following their own dreams and not catering to the needs and wants of everyone around them. What propelled them to hero status was the inner strength and visions they held about themselves.

Are you ready to shake off that niceness? Can you see how your patients could benefit from a nurse who is strong and guided by an inner compass, instead of being guided by the court of public opinion?

List the pros and cons that niceness has had on your career. In other words, what have you gained as a nurse as a result of your niceness? What have you lost?

Pros                                        Cons

_____          _____
_____          _____
_____          _____
_____          _____

Now, imagine that you are no longer a nice nurse. You are a strong nurse guided by your inner compass. You have the qualities that your heroes embody. How would that impact who you are as a nurse? How would that impact the decisions you make? How would it impact your personal life, for instance the modeling it would provide for your children?

Write it down.

_____
_____
_____
_____
_____
_____
_____
_____

Self-care is not a luxury; it is a necessity. It is the ultimate insult to whatever source you believe to be our Creator to not treat yourself as a valuable and valued person. Treat yourself with the respect you give your patients. Advocate for yourself the way you champion your patients. Imagine and create a world where you matter.

# Resources and Bibliography

Morgenstern, J. *Organizing From the Inside Out*. Owl Books. 1998.

National Association for Health and Fitness. Available at: www.physicalfitness.org.

National Institutes of Health. Available at: www.nih.gov.

Orman, S. *The Laws of Money, The Lessons of Life: Keep What You Have and Create What You Deserve*. Free Press. 2003.

Richardson, C. *Take Time for Your Life*. Broadway Books, New York, NY.1998.

Roizen, M. *The RealAge© Makeover: Take Years Off Your Looks and Add Them to Your Life*. Harper Resource. 2004.

The American Dietetic Association. Available at: www.eatright.org.

The Financial Planning Association. Available at www.fpanet.org.

The President's Council on Physical Fitness and Sports. Available at: www.fitness.gov.

The Schools of Coachville. Available at: www.coachville.com.

# Chapter Four

# Take Two Affirmations and Call Me in the Morning

"The future belongs to those who believe in the beauty of their dreams."
Eleanor Roosevelt

A positive attitude is sometimes given a bad rap. Sometimes people see a positive attitude as a Pollyanna approach to life. "Get real!" is often the consensus. But having a positive attitude doesn't mean you live under a rock and are oblivious to the realities of life. It simply means you choose to look at life in a way that benefits you the most.

In this chapter we'll take a look at how to use some powerful and positive tools to move your personal life and your professional career forward in a way that serves you. The tools we'll use include creating a vision, identifying your values, developing a mission statement, and using affirmations. Let's begin

## Creating a Vision

People who have the ability to predict or create a new reality are often referred to as visionaries. They are people who look far beyond what most of us are able to see as they imagine and often create bigger and greater things and a bigger and greater world. People like Albert Einstein, who made the connection between energy and matter with his equation $E=mc^2$; and Martin Luther King, whose vision was for a world where people of color had equal rights; and Steve Jobs, who saw a world where the average person and the computer would meet; and Florence Nightingale, who brought the nursing profession to the world.

Visionaries are what some great people become; vision is what we all have the ability to use. Stephen Covey writes that vision is "the ability to see beyond our present reality, to create, to invent what does not yet exist, to become what we not yet are" (Covey, 1995).

Some of the benefits of creating a vision include:

- Eliminating in-the-box thinking

- Developing a laser-like focus
- Creating an environment that is open to unique solutions
- Identifying direction and purpose
    Used with permission from Education Leadership Toolkit, an online publication at www.nsba.org/sbot/toolkit/index/html. Copyright 1997, National School Boards Association. All rights reserved.

Susan is a new RN, but she isn't new to the health profession. She was raised in a dysfunctional family of limited financial and emotional resources. Few in her family have escaped the family legacy of dysfunction and a life lived on the edges of poverty. But Susan always had a vision in her mind of much more. She graduated from high school and began working as a nursing assistant. Always holding her vision of becoming a psychiatric RN, she worked hard, saved her money, and continued her education – advancing from nursing assistant to LPN to associate RN to a baccalaureate RN. Her vision never wavered. And she is now planning to continue her education to become the psychiatric clinical nurse specialist she dreamed of and help others to develop their own visions.

We all know someone like Susan, who held firmly to a vision greater than the reality they knew. Without that vision there would be little chance that Susan would have become a nurse, let alone escape the legacy of her upbringing.

What vision do you hold for yourself? Take a moment to write down your vision. If you don't have a vision, now is the time to consider developing one. Be specific. What reality do you want to create for yourself? What would it look like? Feel like? Be descriptive.

The vision I hold for myself is

_____
_____
_____


I will know that I have achieved my vision when

_____
_____
_____
_____

**Values**

Everybody has values specific to him or her. Your values may not be the same values that are near and dear to your spouse or friend or colleague. That does not make your values more or less important than someone else's.

Although we all have our individual values that make up who we are, these values are often crushed and compromised by things we think we should do or ought to do, the demands of other people, or the demands of our work environment when it is not in sync with who we are.

It's important to understand what our individual values are because it makes it so much easier to make decisions that reflect those values. According to the coaching program Personal Foundation/Personal Freedom, values bring fulfillment and wants bring gratification (Coachville, 2003). Now on first look, gratification doesn't seem like a bad thing. However, fulfillment is much more satisfying because it fills us up and has lasting value. Living our values is more of a state of being than a destination.

The key is to discover what your values are and then orient your life around them. Understanding your values makes it easier to set goals, create your mission statement, and live a life where you are propelled forward rather than backward or off course entirely.

Take a few moments and select 20 values from this list. Remember, they should be values, not needs, should, wants, or so forth. The values are those words that represent what makes you feel fulfilled and complete.

**ADVENTURE**
Risk
The unknown
Thrill
Danger
Speculation
Dare
Gamble
Endeavor
Quest
Experiment
Exhilaration
Venture

**BEAUTY**
Grace
Refinement
Elegance
Attractiveness
Loveliness
Radiance
Magnificence
Gloriousness
Taste

**TO CATALYZE**
Impact
Move forward
Touch
Turn on
Coach
Spark
Encourage
Influence
Stimulate
Energize
Alter

**TO CREATE**
Design
Invent
Synthesize
Imagination
Ingenuity
Originality
Conceive
Plan
Build
Perfect
Assemble
Inspire

**TO FEEL**
Emote
To experience
Sense
To glow
To feel good
Be with
Energy flow
In touch with
Sensations

**TO CONTRIBUTE**
Serve
Improve
Augment
Endow
Strengthen
Facilitate
Minister to
Grant
Provide
Foster
Assist

**TO DISCOVER**
Learn
Detect
Perceive
Locate
Realize
Uncover
Discern
Distinguish
Observe

**TO LEAD**
Guide
Inspire
Influence
Cause
Arouse
Enroll
Reign
Govern
Rule
Persuade

Encourage
Model

## MASTERY
Expert
Dominate field
Adept
Superiority
Primacy
Preeminence
Greatest
Best
Outdo
Set standards
Excellence

## PLEASURE
Have fun
Be hedonistic
Sex
Sensual
Bliss
Be amused
Play games
Sports

## TO RELATE
Be connected
Part of community
Family
To unite
To nurture
Be linked
Be bonded
Be integrated
Be with

## BE SENSITIVE
Tenderness
Touch
Perceive
Be present
Empathize
Support
Show compassion
Respond
See

## BE SPIRITUAL
Be aware
Be accepting
Be awake
Relate with God
Devoting
Holy
Honoring
Be passionate
Religious

## TO TEACH
Educate
Instruct
Enlighten
Inform
Prepare
Edify
Prime
Uplift
Explain

## TO WIN

Prevail
Accomplish
Attain
Score
Acquire
Win over
Triumph
Predominate
Attract

Take a look at your 20 values. Cross off any that appear to be needs, wants, or shoulds for you. Now narrow the field down to five dominant values. Pick one value and list ten things that you can do to honor that value.

For instance, say that your number one value is to be connected. Some of the ten things you might do to honor that value are: join a professional association, do your exercise in a gym where there are other people rather than walking by yourself, nurture your friendships and make frequent get-togethers, eliminate those activities in your life that make you feel isolated, teach a class, and so forth.

Value #1:_____

10 steps:
1.

2.

3.

4.

5.

6.

7.

8.

9.

10.

After you have fully met that number one value, you can move on to your number two value. By taking these steps you will find that your life is revolving more around your values than the shoulds and needs in your life. You will feel more energized and fulfilled, and definitely more positive.

**Creating a Mission Statement**

A vision statement is the picture we hold in our mind for a larger life than we might currently have. A mission statement is the bylaw you create that moves you toward your vision. Developing a personal mission statement can be a powerful way to focus your attention and energy towards goals that are meaningful to you and achieving them in a way that honors your values. How the mission statement is framed or created is really unimportant. What is important is that it reflects what is important to you and what you value and hope to accomplish.

Mission statements have become popular in the business world where corporations and companies come together to create a statement that reflects who they are and what they hope to accomplish. Unfortunately, many mission statements are just a collection of words that are more an exercise of the public relations department than a collectively held belief system. In cases such as these, the mission statement is not worth the paper it's printed on.

However, a mission statement that is meaningful to the individual and/or the stakeholders becomes a beacon that guides the employer and employee's actions. Any action or decision can then be based on the mission statement. Does this proposed action or decision move me/us closer to or farther away from this mission statement? Asking that question can clear away the data that is clouding your vision and makes the decision that is right for you easier to make. At the very least, a mission statement makes decision-making reflect who you are as a person and what you hold dear and important to you.

When writing your mission statement, keep the following in mind:

- Make the mission statement no longer than two sentences. Any longer and it becomes cumbersome and difficult to remember.

- Write the mission statement to reflect what is important to you, not what you think other people would be interested in.

- Write the mission statement in present tense, as if it is already a done deal. For instance, "I believe in living my life with integrity and passion and helping the people around me to do the same."

- Create the mission statement to reflect the values that are inspiring and important to you. We all have many values. Narrow your values down to the key, overriding values that are nonnegotiable.

Remember Susan? She had a general vision for herself to grow beyond the dysfunctional and poor family she grew up in. And she had a specific vision to become a psychiatric clinical nurse specialist who could help other people in their journey through life. What do you think Susan's mission statement was?

It might have looked something like this: "I continue to honor my love of education and seek opportunities to grow as a person and as a nurse so that I may better help others."

Now it's your turn. You have an idea of what your vision is, now it's time to create a mission statement that reflects that vision and helps to propel you forward.

In one or two sentences, create a mission statement that you can use as your guiding statement in life. Remember that you want to choose one or two values that encompass all your values.

My mission statement is:

_____
_____
_____
_____

Now write your mission statement on some slips of paper and put them where you will see them everyday. A great place is on your bathroom mirror, so you see it at the beginning and end of the day. Another place might be your computer, your car dashboard, or in your wallet. The idea is to subtly plant the mission in your subconscious mind.

For a more in depth look at creating empowering mission statements, a great resource is Appendix A in Stephen Covey's book, *First Things First*. It guides the reader through the mission statement process – assessing strengths, character, what work and family aspects are most valued, and so forth.

## Affirmations

Say the word "affirmations" and many people will think back to the *Saturday Night Live* show and a particular skit where the comedian looked into a mirror and repeated an affirmation to the hoots of the audience. Something along the lines of: "I'm good enough, and heck, people like me!" It gave the idea of affirmations a bad name for a while. But many successful people have used affirmations for years.

An affirmation is simply a sentence spoken in the present tense that reflects what you want to happen or what you want to be. They are written and spoken in the present tense because of the belief that the power of words can indeed create the reality.

Affirmations can be powerful and shore you up in times when you most need it. For instance, you need to give a presentation and are filled with dread at the thought of standing in front of a large audience. You might develop an affirmation just for this occasion. It might be, "I am a competent speaker and the audience is learning and enjoying."

The best way to use affirmations is to make them specific and repeat them often to yourself. In the case of the frightened public speaker above, saying the affirmation once would hardly make a dent in your level of anxiety. However, repeating the affirmation several times a day for a week before the presentation, and then right before walking to the podium, instills the message on a much deeper level.

Words, spoken or written, have great power. We know that words can hurt us; words can also heal us, empower us, and inspire us to do more than we thought possible.

Here are some sample affirmations for happiness and success:

- I choose to put love and joy into everything I do – my positive feelings fill me with the power to succeed.

- I choose to feel happy, therefore I AM happy!

- My continuous success springs from my own well – I am positive and joyful every day of my life.

- I accept that the greater my successes, the greater my ability I have to share my knowledge with others.

- I am the creator of my successes and my happiness. I am therefore happy and successful every day of my life, because I choose it.

- I am aware that my success and happiness is a direct result of my positive thoughts, words, actions, and feelings.

- I choose to surround myself with positive and happy people.

- I am happy for others when they succeed. We are all one, and another's success is mine as well.
  With permission from Your Daily Affirmation, available at http://www.yourdailyaffirmation.com.

Do you see how the affirmations above are framed as if they are already true? That is the power of affirmations. To act, as if it is so. To do, as if it is so. To be, as if it is so. Many successful people swear by the power of affirmations.

What affirmation would add to the quality of your life? How might a busy day on your surgical floor look if you had an affirmation to help you? For instance, "I am helping my patients and handling each crisis competently."

How about dealing with your children? "I am a thoughtful and loving parent and I am teaching my children to be thoughtful and loving as well." Your turn. Take a few moments and experiment with some affirmations that might inspire you.

I am

_____

_____

I am

_____

_____

I am

_____

_____

I am

_____

_____

Remember to repeat these affirmations – out loud – at least several times a day. Saying your affirmation in the morning is a great way to get the day off to a great start. You can also post your affirmations, much like you do your mission statement, in places where you'll see it and be able to reflect on it.

# Resources and Bibliography

Covey, Stephen. *First Things First*. Fireside; New York, NY.1995.

National School Boards Association, National Science Foundation grant. Available at: www.nsba.org/sbot/toolkit/cav.html.

Leonard, Thomas. *The Portable Coach*. Scribner; New York, NY:1998.

Personal Freedom Program. Coachville.com. 2000-2003.

Your Daily Affirmation. Available at: www.yourdailyaffirmation.com.

# Chapter Five

# The Use of Restraints

"To move freely you must be deeply rooted."
Bella Lewitzky

T he use of restraints is fraught with debate – does it keep the patient safe from harm, or does it so restrict freedom of movement as to be considered potentially harmful? The answer is – yes.

The same can be said about restraints in our lives. Restraints can keep us safe – think seatbelts, for instance. On the other hand, we can be harmed by anything that restricts our freedom to be who and what we are. Two examples of such restraints are boundaries and the toxic work environment. We can be injured or hurt when someone violates our boundaries with either actions or words. And a toxic work environment has a way of seeping into our personal lives as we fret away our free time dreading the return to "that place."

Let's explore the ideas of how boundaries and a toxic workplace can restrain and restrict you.

## Boundaries

You feel taken advantage of – used and abused. No one understands you. You get all the difficult patient assignments. You're the one always asked to work an extra shift. You're the one who is the emotional punching bag of that screaming physician.

At home, things are not much better. You're the one asked to run the school bake sale, coach the 12-and-under soccer team, and plan that fundraiser – again. You wonder if you have a sign on your back that says, "Kick me – hard."

It's no accident that some people are consistently taken advantage of and feel that their coworkers, friends, and family seem to not honor or respect them. If this sounds eerily familiar to you, it's quite possible that you, like many other people, have boundary issues.

Boundary issues are nothing to sniff at. Countries have gone to war over some imaginary line on the ground, some boundary that each side believes is the line of demarcation separating one from the other. Boundaries tell the world, This is where I start and you leave off.

And nurses certainly understand the idea of defending boundaries for their patients and protecting them from unwanted visitors or an ill-timed procedure. They understand the value and importance of keeping the patient safe, intact, and secure. But what about nurses protecting their own boundaries? For many nurses, the idea of protecting their boundaries – of even understanding where their boundaries are – is not on their radar screen.

Nurses are so vigilant about protecting and caring and advocating for others, that the line of demarcation becomes obscured and blurred. Their boundaries barely exist and sometimes cease to exist. And any time your boundaries are weak, so too is your self-esteem. Without strong boundaries, you are not a strong individual; you are merely an extension of everyone else in your life. You're there for them – and missing in action for yourself.

Before we go any farther and you begin setting boundaries for others, it's important to honestly assess your role in any situation. Do your words or actions play any part in the situation? In other words, do you communicate cleanly and let the other person know that you've been hurt or offended? Do you give the person you believe is hurting you in some way an opportunity to explain and/or apologize in private? Ask yourself, Am I somehow participating in this situation? Before you start setting boundaries, it's only fair that you are sure that you're not stepping over someone else's line.

## What are boundaries?

Boundaries are those lines we draw in the sand to define who we are, and to protect us from real or perceived harm. These imaginary lines are drawn around our hearts, minds, souls, and even our bodies.

Firm boundaries are all about honoring and respecting yourself enough to tell the world, "I am an intelligent, compassionate person, and I am worthy of your respect. And I think enough of myself to make sure that I am respected." This is a message nurses need to hear. You are in the business of caring and treating patients; of advocating and honoring your patients. But if nurses don't do that for themselves, they are only paying lip service to the idea that the profession deserves respect. Understand this – if you don't respect yourself as an individual first, then you have no right to expect anyone else to respect you or the nursing profession.

The important thing to keep in mind is that boundaries, and setting boundaries, are a purely subjective and personal thing. Only you can determine what your boundaries are, how you want them to look, and what consequence you will use if someone violates them. Determining how you want your boundaries to be is an important part in defining who you are as a person. And strong boundaries will improve the quality of your life, because you will learn to not tolerate the things that do not add to the quality of your life.

Most of us have strong boundaries when it comes to not permitting unwanted sexual advances, inappropriate touching, or physical abuse. You may also prefer that others not "invade your personal space" by standing too close. It's worth noting that the size of someone's personal space may have a lot to do with cultural beliefs – some cultures are more reserved and require a much larger physical boundary, while other cultures feel more comfortable with physical contact and prefer a smaller boundary. Neither is wrong because physical boundaries are all about what makes you comfortable.

Here are a few boundary scenarios that may sound familiar:

The nurse manager who frequently asks you to cover for another nurse, Nellie No Show, and appeals to your feelings of guilt by counting all the ways she goes above and beyond as a nurse manager.

Then there's Dr. Iknoweverything, who shrugs off your clinical observations with a wave of the hand and has honed his ability to make you feel small in front of patients to an art form.

Or the 'friend' who seems to always know when you are spending alone time to work on your hobby, and has a knack for interrupting that precious time with the crisis du jour.

Remember, you are always teaching others how to treat you. Every time you allow yourself to be disrespected, you are teaching others that their behavior is acceptable. Conversely, when you quietly and firmly bring someone's attention to the fact that they are being disrespectful or not honoring your boundaries, you are telling that person, and the world, that you will not tolerate such behavior. So, what are you teaching others about how you want to be treated?

## Weak boundaries

It may be true that opposites attract, but it is more true that like attracts like. If your boundaries are weak, take a good look around, because people who disrespect and violate your boundaries probably surround you. Why not? You're easy picking. Weak boundaries attract needy or disrespectful people. The nurse with weak boundaries can't say no.

"Jane, can you work another double?"
"Steve, you don't mind heading that team again, do you?"
"Sally, can you take the next (your fifth) admission?"

The nurse with weak boundaries reluctantly says okay while her internal organs twist into a mangled mass of self-loathing. "Why did I say yes? I hate this job." It's hard to look yourself in the mirror. You caved in – again. You wonder, "Where's my spine?"

However, the nurse with strong boundaries sends a clear message to everyone that she has respect and a higher level of self-esteem. She has more energy because she doesn't operate from a position of fear. That's because strong boundaries help you grow emotionally and developmentally. You attract like-minded, strong people. Your communication with others comes from a place that honors you, and therefore, honors others.

## Why do we have weak boundaries?

Sometimes weak boundaries are the result of guilt – the gift that keeps on giving. The type of guilt that causes weak boundaries is based on a belief that you don't deserve to make yourself important in your own life. You worry what other people will think about you, and that's a game you just can't win. The good news is that other people don't have the luxury of thinking about you 24/7/365. They've got their own lives to worry about.

Difficulty saying no is a large reason nurses have weak boundaries. Think of two-year-olds and their reputation for the terrible "no's". Saying no is a developmental phase that is a critical piece to their development as individuals. The two-year-old makes her thoughts and desires known as she is discovering them. If that developmental phase is crushed, you have a child who may never develop a strong sense of self. The same is true for the adult. Saying no – developing those boundaries – is an important part of refining and developing the individual.

Some people have a high toleration level. Now, that might sound good – for instance, the patient with a high tolerance to pain is often regarded in a more positive light than the individual with a low tolerance. But in reality, a high toleration level does not serve us well. It means we need an extraordinary amount of pain inflicted upon us before we respond to negative behavior from people or a particular situation. That can't be good! Consequently, we may be taken advantage of, taken for granted, and even mistreated for quite some time before we feel compelled to say enough is enough.

We live in a world where we are constantly overstimulated – e-mail, faxes, PDAs, cell phones, computers, work lives, personal lives, families – our brains and bodies are taking in millions of bits of information all the time. We get so busy we don't notice when one of our boundaries is violated. Or, we just don't have the psychic or emotional energy to point out that we notice our boundary has been violated and deal with it. We've been desensitized and have become too numb and exhausted to react.

And of course, low self-esteem is a sure formula for weak boundaries. We don't deserve (or so we think) to be treated as well as we'd like. We become an easy mark for passive-aggressive compliments or intimidating behavior aimed at keeping us in our place and controlling our behavior. Someone with low self-esteem and weak boundaries becomes a sure foil for those people who want to improve the quality of their lives at your expense.

## How do I set up strong boundaries?

The first step is to decide what your boundaries are now. What are your physical boundaries? Spiritual boundaries? Creative boundaries? Emotional boundaries? Mental boundaries? Financial boundaries? Are you happy with some and not others?

Now decide how far you want to extend or expand your boundaries. For instance, if you are uncomfortable greeting people with a hug and instead prefer to shake hands, decide if that is your hard and fast boundary and what the exceptions might be. Be clear in your mind exactly what you want your boundaries to look like so that you can more easily define those boundaries to others.

Step three is to clue people in that your boundaries have changed. Let people know that you may have accepted a particular behavior in the past, but that it is no longer the case. When you expand your boundaries, it impacts other people in your life, so it's only fair to give them a warning. Deliver news of your new boundaries with tact and clarity. Practice your tone of voice, stance, and facial expression, since all of these also deliver a message. You want to be respectful and firm. Think about writing down your boundary and placing it in a place where you will see it everyday. Then, when you've mastered one boundary you can move on to the next.

You might say, "It makes me uncomfortable (or whatever word describes how you feel) when you make comments about my appearance. I've decided that I don't want to hear those comments anymore, and I ask you not to comment about my appearance again."

Or, "It makes me uncomfortable when you touch me like that. Please do not do that again."

The final step is to decide how you will enforce your boundaries when someone tests your resolve – and they will! What will the consequence be? Because the fact is, some people who offend your boundaries are more than happy to do so. They need a reminder when they overstep the mark, and they need a consequence that will help them step back and reconsider their actions or words. Pick a consequence that you feel confident you can follow through on. If you fail to follow through with a consequence you have again taught others how you expect to be treated.

People are used to behaving around you in a certain way. They will probably say they understand, but will test the waters to see if you are committed to upholding these changes. You will need to repeat your boundary statement over and over and then decide at what point you will issue the ultimatum. Do not over explain your boundaries. You need only repeat the boundary statement. When you over explain, you give the other person the right to negotiate what your boundaries should be. That decision is only yours to make.

> Example: " I've asked you twice not to discredit me in front of a patient. If you do it again I will speak to the nurse manager (or the ultimatum of your choosing)."

You are the one who decides what the ultimatum will be, and you must be willing to follow through. If you don't, you are allowing your boundaries to be violated even though you've explicitly made it clear that it makes you unhappy. And obviously the person violating your boundaries cares nothing about your feelings.

How do you know your boundaries have been violated? If the violation is not obvious to you, your body will give you clues. You may experience a visceral reaction as if someone punched you in the stomach, or you may feel humiliated, angry, guilty, or disappointed. You might wonder, How could he say or do that to me? People with passive-aggressive behavior can do or say something to us that violates our boundary, yet we feel confused by our feelings. That person is smiling at me, so why do I feel so horrible? Well, my friend, you better check your back because you're probably bleeding! You've been dealt a blow. Learn to trust your gut. It's a survival mechanism that we experience for a reason. Don't intellectualize too much. Get out of your head where the "shoulds" live and into your body where your intuition – that visceral intelligence we all have – will clue you in.

People in public safety often advise women to honor and listen to their gut feelings before stepping into an elevator with a stranger. The women who end up as victims in these situations are the ones who ignore their gut feelings that something doesn't feel right by intellectualizing the situation – he's dressed nicely, or, I'll hurt his feelings if I don't get on the elevator. Those gut feelings about the stranger in the elevator, or the gut feeling that the patient in room 243 is going to crash even when all clinical signs point otherwise, are a form of intuition or higher intelligence that is a part of our biology. Learning to silence that visceral intelligence is a mistake. The same is true of the gut feeling you get when dealing with the passive-aggressive person. On the surface everything seems fine, but your body doesn't lie to you. The passive-aggressive person is deliberate in their intentions, even as they smile at you.

Recall a time when you're boundaries were violated. How did it make you feel? Make your writing as descriptive as possible so you really get in touch with the feeling you experienced and can more easily identify it if it happens again.

_____
_____
_____
_____
_____
_____

Now make a list of boundaries you are no longer willing to have violated. It's no longer okay for other people to:

_____
_____
_____
_____
_____
_____
_____

Now let's look at some language to help you defend your boundaries. Once you get an idea of how the language works, you can easily adjust it to fit most situations. Remember, make your boundaries specific and make your consequence clear and do-able.

**Setting the boundary:** "When you yell at me in front of a patient, it undermines my professionalism. I ask that you speak to me in private and as professional to professional."

**Repeating the boundary:** "I have already spoken to you about yelling at me in front of a patient."

**Warning the offender:** "Please do not do that again or I will need to walk away/go to administration/report you."

**Action/consequence:** "You are yelling. I will take this up with administration."

Decide on a boundary you wish to strengthen.
Set the boundary:
_____
_____

Repeat the boundary:
_____
_____
_____
_____

Your warning:
_____
_____
_____
_____

Your
consequence:_____

The key to any situation that revolves around boundary issues is to think about what you want to convey, say it respectfully and firmly, and then absolutely carry it through. Always keep your voice calm and collected. If you are not prepared to see this through to the end, you will seriously jeopardize your credibility.

Once you feel confident about your ability to set your boundaries and to uphold them, you'll begin to see how it relates to other aspects of your life. Remember that every interaction you have with family, friends, coworkers, your boss, and even the grocery clerk is an opportunity to enhance the quality of your life or diminish it.

## Mistakes to avoid

Okay, so you want to create stronger boundaries. I must warn you first that there are some pitfalls to avoid. One mistake people make is setting the boundaries too low. They feel uncomfortable extending their boundaries too much, and they become nervous about stepping on toes or making anyone else uncomfortable. However, if the thought of extending your boundary doesn't make you a bit nervous, it's probably not big enough. It's important to step outside of your comfort zone a bit. Then again, don't set your boundaries too high. If your boundaries are too high, they become difficult to enforce and uphold. To get your feet wet, try setting firmer boundaries with people who are not close to you, for instance acquaintances or colleagues you don't work closely with at work. Family, friends, coworkers, and bosses may seem too intimidating at first. It helps to have some successes under your belt before you begin setting firm boundaries with the people who are closest to you.

Don't argue with other people about your boundaries. There are occasions when it makes more sense to walk away from the situation than to become too defensive about a boundary. Anytime you get into a debate or argument about what your boundaries should or should not be, you are essentially giving your power away. You are allowing others to negotiate what your boundaries should be. It's like handing your life over to others and saying, "Here's my life. Decide what I should do and get back to me on it."

Above all, remember that your boundaries are solely for the purpose of upholding and protecting who you are. Don't use it to try and control the behavior of others. Setting boundaries is all about you, not the other person.

## The Toxic Work Environment

You're off for two days, yet part of your mind is already dreading the return to 'that place.' Just thinking about it, you feel your pulse quicken and your neck muscles tense up. The nurse manager plays favorites, the patient assistants seem to conspire against you and against doing their job, the unit is short-staffed and under-resourced, and that's just for starters. Welcome to the toxic work environment.

The healthcare world does not have the monopoly on toxic work environments. It's old hat for the business and corporate world. Many of us are familiar with the *Dilbert* cartoon that satirizes and pokes fun at the craziness that invades the workplace. Still, nurses expect the healthcare workplace to be patient-driven and nurse-friendly, with a compassion-focused mission. Instead they discover, that in some cases, healthcare is first and foremost a business with insecure people (think *Dilbert*) scrambling and bidding for power while the PR people put a 'because we care' spin on the fallout. Sometimes it's not pretty, and nurses who practice in these settings feel particularly betrayed. In situations such as these, the toxic environment usually exists up and down the ladder. Each layer of the organization is diseased.

In other settings, the toxic environment may extend to one or more people who taint the workplace. It may be the nurse who intimidates her colleagues and her patients with bullying-type behavior. Or it may be the surgeon who has a loose grasp on her anger, causing nurses and other physicians to feel off balance and tense in the OR. These situations hold the rest of the staff hostage to the whims and demands of the toxic coworker. Everyone gives in to get by. (For toxic relationships, see chapter two)

Sometimes you might be the only person at your workplace that experiences a toxic work environment. It might be that a nurse colleague is jealous of your skill level or your standing on the unit, or your boss may feel threatened by your skills and ability to lead because she believes that it threatens to reveal the areas where she is lacking. For the nurse on the receiving end of a toxic boss, work can be a less-than-desirable place to practice.

Toxicity in the work setting is quickly gaining national attention, specifically when it comes to bullying behavior – whether it's the bully coworker or a bully boss. Much of the attention has grown out of the bully-type behavior of children and the sometimes tragic and violent results that have played before our eyes on television and the newspapers.

The Campaign Against Workplace Bullying is a nonprofit education research and advocacy program that began in 1998. The website, The

Workplace Bullying and Trauma Institute, available at www.bullybusters.org, is considered to be a national clearinghouse for learning about bullying and has provided advice and resources to victims of bullying behavior. Authors and founders of the campaign, Gary Namie, PhD, and Ruth Namie, PhD, write in their book that the #1 reason for being bullied is the "Target's refusal to be subservient, to not go along with being controlled," and the #2 reason is "'Bully Envy'" of the Target's skill, knowledge, or ability to work with people (Namie and Namie, 40, 41, 2000)." The good news, according to the authors, is that good employers get rid of bullies. The bad news is...you guessed it, bad employers promote the bullies.

Bullying in the workplace is not good for you – emotionally or physically. The symptoms of stress indicate trauma – physical symptoms of stress, thinking-cognitive symptoms, and emotional symptoms. According to the Campaign Against Workplace Bullying, some of the effects of bullying are (Namie and Namie, 61, 2000):

1. Stress, anxiety
2. Depression
3. Exhaustion
4. Insecurity, self-doubt
5. Shame, embarrassment, guilt

Dr. Judith Briles has written frequently on the role saboteurs play in the toxic workplace. She says that it's important to identify the saboteur that may lurk around your work site. A saboteur is a person who undermines or destroys someone's personal or professional integrity, life or credibility, or damages someone's self-worth or self-esteem.

Want to know if there is a saboteur in your midst? Briles has identified 12 scenarios:

1. Does anyone feel that her (or his) job is in jeopardy?
2. Does anyone routinely deny involvement in certain activities, yet know all the details?
3. Does anyone constantly realign their friendships?
4. Does anyone encourage gossip?
5. Does anyone keep a tally sheet?
6. Does information pass you by?
7. Is anyone on your team excessively helpful?
8. Does anyone stand to profit by another's mistake?

9.  Does anyone bypass your authority or go over your head?
10. Does anyone encourage others to take on tasks that appear impossible?
11. Does anyone take credit for another's work done?
12. Does anyone discount another's contributions?
    Used with permission. *Zapping Conflict in the Health Care Workplace*(c) 2003 by Judith Briles, www.Briles.com.

Briles writes that saboteurs are usually exposed as time goes by, but that it's still important to stay out of their line of fire, document, and when necessary, confront the person.

If you are being bullied at work, you must take action. That action may include confronting the bully, notifying supervisors up the chain of command, filing a complaint, taking legal action, or leaving the job. Bullying behavior in the workplace – especially if the bully is your boss – is a serious toxic situation and the implications of this situation are beyond the scope of this book. You may need to seek professional (attorney, professional organizations such as the Campaign Against Workplace Bullying, or counselor) to help to sort out your feelings and put a plan into effect that will protect you. Resources for dealing with a bully in the workplace are listed at the end of this chapter.

If the entire culture of the workplace is diseased and toxic, it may be in your best interest to cut your losses, walk away, and find another job (see chapter seven). Such an environment needs a total overhaul, and you could spend a lifetime tilting at windmills and never make a dent. The question to ask yourself is, "What do I gain by staying?" I've talked to a number of nurses who worked in such environments, but opted to stay. Their reasons:

> "I've been here too long to leave."
> "I'm too old to find another job."
> "It's so convenient and close to where I live."
> "It's probably the same every other place."

My response to that:
> "Are you going for the merit badge in suffering?"
> "You'll be the same age no matter what you do."
> "Expand your horizons."
> "Can you spell R-A-T-I-O-N-A-L-I-Z-A-T-I-O-N?"

If your work environment is causing you more pain than you would like, you have arrived at a fork in the road. It's time to make a decision. The problem is either fixable or it's not. If it's fixable, you can work toward making your workplace a more collaborative environment. This might involve going through the appropriate channels of authority to voice your concern, or it might mean setting firm boundaries with the offender and dealing with the offender in a direct manner:

> "Sally, when you second guess my clinical skills it makes me feel as if you don't trust my judgment. Can we discuss this and clear the air?"

Bear in mind that if Sally is a true bully, she won't care about your feelings, and she'll probably respond in a negative manner. But, you'll have put your cards on the table by confronting her in a nonjudgmental manner. In other words, you'll know where you stand. Oftentimes, just making a point of dealing directly with the offending individual is enough to let them know that you're on to them and that you have the courage to confront them. Bullies often like to pick on people they perceive as easy targets. With that said, some bullies deliberately target strong individuals who threaten them – either with their knowledge, reputation, or leadership skills.

What happens if your boss is the toxic one? You can try the direct approach above; just remember to keep your voice and body language neutral and nonaccusatory.

> "Nancy, lately I'm feeling that I'm given the more difficult patient assignments, and I appreciate your faith in me. Is there some way we can give some of the other nurses an opportunity to gain some more experience in dealing with difficult patients?"

Do you see how the wording of the question leaves Nancy a back door? You haven't pushed her up against a wall by saying, "It's not fair. You're giving me all the work." When you push someone like Nancy up against the wall, you're more likely to suffer a fate far worse than a difficult patient assignment. She has the power to make your job miserable. However, by framing the question in a collaborative, we're-all-here-for-the-patient point of view, you give Nancy the opportunity to be the good guy and use her power to boot! That's called a win-win situation. Nevertheless, if Nancy makes it clear that she'll continue doing what she's doing because she says so – you may need to decide if that's a situation you can live with or if you want to take the issue up with her boss.

Sometimes the situation is not fixable, and you still have a choice – you can begin again in another unit or another facility. That is the take-away message in

77

all of this. You always have a choice – about taking action and how you choose to perceive the situation. That's where the power is. The choices are in your hands.

Stop for a moment and take stock of your workplace environment. Here are some questions that may help you decide if your workplace is toxic for you.

For the most part, when I am at work I feel (describe in detail).

_____

_____

_____

_____

For the most part, my coworkers add the following to my practice and my life.

_____

_____

_____

For the most part, my boss
adds_____

_____

_____to my practice and my life.

I feel supported and valued in the workplace. True or False? _____

If I had it to do over again, I would

_____

_____

For the most part, I believe I am making a positive difference. True or False?_____

I am respected and supported at work. True or False? _____

I feel that my job is a good fit for me. True or False? _____

How did you do? Any surprises? Perhaps you've realized that you would be better off in another workplace environment that provides a healthier place for you to practice. To guide you through the process of moving on, read chapter seven "Calling the Code."

If you pay attention to these restraints in your life – the boundaries and toxic work environment – you'll have the freedom to live a life you design and a career that you create. Someone once said that it is better to die on your feet than to live on your knees. Ask yourself, Where are you living?

# Resources and Bibliography

Adams, S. *Dilbert and the Way of the Weasel.* HarperCollins. New York, NY:2002.

Briles, J. *Zapping Conflict in the Health Care Workplace©.*Available at: www.Briles.com.

Coachville. Available at: www.coachville.com.

Information website. Available at: www.kickbully.com.

Leonard, T. *The Portable Coach.* Scribner; New York, NY:1998.

Lichtenberg, R. *Work Would Be Great If It Weren't for the People.* Hyperion; New York, NY:1998.

Namie, G & Namie, R. *The Bully at Work: What You Can Do to Stop the Hurt and Reclaim Your Dignity.* Sourcebooks, Inc.IL:2000.

Reinhold, S. *Toxic Work.* Penguin; New York, NY:1996.

The Campaign Against Workplace Bullying and the Workplace Bullying and Trauma Institute. Available at: www.bullybusters.org

# Chapter Six

# Breathe Life Into Your Career

"The only place you find success before work is in the dictionary."
May V. Smith

Sometimes we may think our career is on a downward spiral, burning and crashing to the ground. The fact is, often times our careers just need to be resuscitated a bit and awakened so that our career is fresh and exciting again.

It's important to give yourself the gift of occasionally breathing life into your career because you deserve a career that excites you and makes you feel fulfilled. Some ways to do that include developing leadership skills, defining success – one person's definition is not necessarily another's – embracing your expertness, and being open to the various practice areas that exist in nursing.

## Follow Your STAR!©

There's no doubt that passion fuels success. It's a natural combination when you think about it. It's so much easier to give your all to something that fuels you and that you love. Conversely, it's much easier to resent giving so much of yourself to something that doesn't add quality to your life.

A formula I have developed – STAR© – is one tool to use for success. Here it is:

S – Success on your own terms
T – True North as your guide
A – Assess and understand who you are
R – Risk it all (within reason, of course!)

Let's break the formula down.

**S – Success on your own terms**. One of the biggest mistakes many of us make is to pursue success based on someone else's definition. What success means to you and what it means to your colleague are usually two very different things. Yet many of us spend much of our lives charging down the path of someone else's life, rather than understanding what path is ours to pursue.

For example, many nurses have been "complimented" by a loved one or even a patient or patient's family member who wondered why a smart woman/man would pursue nursing and not medicine. This is a prime example of someone/society's definition of success. Every family has its own definition of success that is overtly or covertly communicated to each family member, such as the parents who are Ivy League professors and define success as someone who follows a similar path. If one of their children decided to become a rap star, that would most likely not fall within the parameters of success.

Rather than follow someone else's definition of success and listen to the "you shoulds" and "you ought to's," we might be better served to understand what success means to us.

Take a moment and think about what success in your career looks like. What does it feel like? Then complete this sentence:

"I know I will be successful when I've/I'm:

_____

_____

_____

_____

**T – True North guiding you**. Navigate life with your inner compass. Keep your decisions centered on your values. It's all about understanding where your True North is. In boating, the captain must know the difference between True North from compass north, which is influenced by the earth's magnetic pull. In life, we must know the difference between our values and the magnetic pull of the "shoulds" and the "ought to's". When we follow True North, we follow a path that is unique to us and make decisions that are right for us.

For example, Sally is a dynamite ICU nurse with impeccable critical care skills. But her True North is calling her to labor and delivery. She's passionate about babies and the birthing process. But her compass north argues that 1) she's got such great critical care skills and she can't just waste them, and 2) what will everyone think if she leaves the prestigious ICU setting? Sally won't find success on her terms until she follows True North to labor and delivery. And moving to L&D may be just a stepping stone toward her ultimate career success – part of a greater plan she can't see yet.

82

**A – Assess and understand who you are**. It's important to understand your strengths and how you can leverage those strengths to take your career to the next level. But first we have to know what those strengths are. Generally a good way to figure out what your true strengths are is to ask trusted and respected colleagues – "In my practice, what do you see as my strengths?" You might also ask your direct supervisor for an honest assessment of your strengths – "Nancy, I want to continue to improve my skills and I respect and value your opinion. What do you see as my strengths?"

For instance, one of your strengths might be that you are technologically savvy and comfortable with any high-tech equipment. How could you leverage that strength? Maybe by providing an inservice for your colleagues to make them feel comfortable and competent with equipment. Or you could improve a piece of equipment or possibly invent an adapter to some equipment that would improve patient outcomes or make the equipment more user friendly.

Perhaps one of your strengths is extraordinary clinical skills. You might leverage that strength by teaching others, writing a "how-to" article on some aspect of patient care, or you might even write a book.

Take a moment and reflect on some of your strengths. What ways could you leverage your strengths in your practice?

_____
_____
_____
_____
_____
_____
_____

It's also important to understand what your weaknesses are and how you might improve some of them. By nature, some of us are more likely to cite a laundry list of weaknesses we believe we possess, while others are more likely to have a more difficult time even considering the possibility that they might have a weakness! I suspect that nurses tend to fall in the first category. So just like your strengths, you might consider asking trusted colleagues or your immediate supervisor for an honest assessment of your weaknesses.

Once you know what your true weaknesses are, you are in a better position to improve upon them. For instance, if your computer skills are a weakness, you might take a computer course, study a computer manual or book, or have a colleague who is skilled with a computer work with you to improve your skills.

Quickly list your strengths and weaknesses.

| Strengths | Weaknesses |
| --- | --- |
| 1. | 1. |
| 2. | 2. |
| 3. | 3. |
| 4. | 4. |
| 5. | 5. |
| 6. | 6. |
| 7. | 7. |
| 8. | 8. |
| 9. | 9. |
| 10. | 10. |

Before you take your list as the ultimate list of your strengths and weaknesses, test them. Compare your list with the input you received from colleagues and supervisors. Their responses may surprise you and buoy your spirits. We're often far too critical of ourselves, while others see us in much more favorable light.

**R – Risk it all (within reason, of course!).** When we push the envelope a bit and push ourselves farther than what we believe we are capable of, we greatly increase the chances of achieving success and growing as a person. We are daring to be great. It doesn't mean we will always succeed, but playing it safe will ultimately hold us back. Remember, Babe Ruth had to strike out many times for each home run.

What ways can you take risks to increase your chances of success in your career? You might give a speech on the use of seat belts to a community group, or you might speak to other nurses about a program on your unit that has decreased the rate of restraints. Or you might consider writing an article for a lay publication or your nursing journal. Then again, you might shadow a nurse who practices in an area that you are really interested in.

If I weren't afraid, I would consider taking the following risks to enhance my career:

---

---

---

---

---

What's holding you back? What steps could you take to eliminate your fear of taking those risks?

## Leadership at the Bedside or in the Board Room

Without a doubt, nurses use leadership skills everyday. But many times, nurses don't recognize their own role as a leader. The staff nurse looks to the nurse manager as the leader, who looks to the nurse executive, who looks to the chief nursing officer or nursing VP, who looks to the president and hospital board as the leaders. While that's how the leadership chain of command works, it doesn't diminish the leadership nurses demonstrate in their roles. Stephen Covey refers to leadership and its "circle of influence" – that we are all leaders with our own circle of influence (Covey, 1995).

It's true that the nursing VP has a larger circle of influence than the nurse manager or the staff nurse, but the impact of that nurse manager or staff nurse's leadership on his or her circle of influence is just as important. As Covey writes, "We may not be *the* leader, but we're *a* leader"(Covey, 1995).

Understand that you are a leader wherever you practice. You use leadership skills as you guide patients and their families through the healthcare system, through a recovery, or toward a good and peaceful death. And those leadership skills are what your patients and their families look to you for. It doesn't matter your patient's status. He or she is vulnerable and looks to you to light the path and guide the way.

Whether we are the leader in a situation or the follower (i.e., team player), we are still powerful because even as a follower we can exhibit leadership. And often during our career we flip/flop between a leadership and a follower-ship role. The reason? Because no matter what role we assume, we are always influencing others. In fact, we cannot not influence people. It's just human nature.

So what are the qualities that signal a good leader? Here are a few:

- Passion. People are naturally drawn to the person with charisma, and that charisma is often driven by that person's passion for what he or she does or believes in. If you are passionate about your practice, people will naturally be drawn to you and want to follow you.

- Students of success. A successful leader is an expert on success. When something goes right, she studies it – why did it work? How can I replicate that? What can I learn from this? Unsuccessful leaders study failure – why did it happen? How can I avoid that again? While it's not a bad thing to understand how to avoid a similar mistake, the problem in studying failure is that you become an expert in – failure! However, if your focus is on success, the rate of failure will naturally diminish. Much like tending a garden, focus on the care of the flowers, and the garden will be even more beautiful and the weeds will decrease on their own.

- Surround yourself with smarter people. A true leader is not afraid of creative and intelligent subordinates. The true leader understands that leadership is a reciprocal relationship. An intelligent and creative staff moves the leadership team and the objective forward. However, the false or ineffective leader is so concerned with watching her back so that none of her staff appear too intelligent or creative, that she misses her objective entirely. Remember, you have to look forward to succeed!

- Communicate cleanly. Say what you mean and mean what you say. Never assume that people understand what you are saying. Ask for feedback. "Sandy, can you give me some feedback on what I just said?" If Sandy can't articulate what you said, you need to clarify. Communicating cleanly with your written and spoken words will make sure that others know when and how to follow you.

Let's take a look at some self-assessment questions you can ask yourself regarding your leadership skills. Answer yes or no. If you answer no, ask yourself how you might develop that skill.

1. Do I see problems as opportunities?
2. Do I know how to set priorities that make sense?
3. Am I courageous in my decision-making?
4. Can I tolerate ambiguity?

5. Do I have a positive attitude toward change?
6. Do I communicate my values?
7. Can I inspire others toward a shared vision?
8. Can I see the "big picture" questions and ask, "what if..."?
9. Can I develop and implement action plans?
10. Do I use goal-setting?
11. Do I encourage dreaming and out-of-the box thinking?
12. Am I a critical and creative thinker?

> Used with permission from Education Leadership Toolkit, an online publication at www.nsba.org/sbot/toolkit/index/html. Copyright 1997, National School Boards Association. All rights reserved.

Dr. Sylvia Rimm wrote two books on successful women and why they are the way they are. Her first book, *See Jane Win*, was the result of data collected from more than 1,000 successful women to determine what factors helped them fulfill their potential. Her second book, *How Jane Won*, interviews 55 successful women from different walks of life and occupations to share their personal paths to success. Interesting to note, two of the 55 women are nurses – Jeanette Ives Erickson, RN, MS, senior vice president of patient care services and chief of nursing for Massachusetts General Hospital; and Pauline Robitaillie, RN, MSN, CNOR, director of surgical services for New England Baptist Hospital.

Rimm's findings from *See Jane Win* include (Rimm, 2001):

1. Girls grow through healthy competition.
2. Girls who see themselves as smart are poised to succeed.
3. All-girl independent or parochial schools can be good choices.
4. Peers matter, for better or worse.
5. Travel has a broadening influence.
6. Successful women had supportive parents.
7. Birth order may not matter, but siblings do.
8. Opportunities spring from obstacles.
9. Successful women have a passion for their work.
10. Balancing work and family life is an ongoing challenge.

> Used with permission, Sylvia Rimm, PhD.

The results of Rimm's study is not lost because we're grown and we can't go back and create a new childhood. The information is important for two reasons – 1) to help us prepare our daughters for the future, and 2) because it may be too late for another childhood, but it's not too late to assimilate the above list and integrate it into our lives.

Take Sandy, for instance. Sandy is pushing 50-years-old. Her childhood never included competition of any kind. She never participated in group activities. Consequently, the idea of competition has never felt comfortable to her. In fact, she sees competition as a negative quality that is the exact opposite of her desire to be a team player.

To make use of competition as a growth factor in her success, perhaps Sandy could join some group activities that involve competition – for example, join a women's softball or volleyball league, or take part in her child's school spelling bee for parents and community members. The idea is that becoming involved in healthy competition would open Sandy's eyes to the value of competition and perhaps make her more comfortable with the idea of stepping outside the comfort of the team player role all the time.

## Are You an Expert?

Here's the deal. There is probably no other profession that runs from accepting its own expertness as quickly as nursing does. Think about it. Most other professions graduate from college still wet behind the ears, diploma in hand, and immediately consider and advertise themselves as experts.

An exaggeration? No. Who in his or her right mind would ever consider using the services of someone who didn't claim to be an expert? Would you consider having that hernia repaired by a surgeon who said, "Well, I'm not really an expert at this, but I'll give it a shot."?

Would you have your taxes done by an accountant who wasn't an expert? "I'm not really an expert, but I'll throw some numbers together." Your car fixed by a mechanic who wasn't an expert? "I'm not really an expert, but let me tinker under the hood for a few minutes."

Do you get the picture? If you practice nursing – you are an expert. You are an expert in your area of practice. Yet for some reason nurses have an unusually hard time claiming their expertness, and many healthcare facilities (acute and chronic) miss a large marketing opportunity by not taking advantage of the collective expert nursing care their facility offers. Smart facilities shout it from the rooftops. They want their communities to know that the nursing care within their walls is expert care aimed at delivering the best outcomes for every patient who enters through those doors.

Remember, humility does not serve the nursing profession and it certainly does not serve you. Practice a few statements to help reflect the expertness you bring to your practice. You might think about how another professional you know (i.e., accountant, teacher, physical therapist) might define his or her expertness. For instance, you might say, "I am a pediatric nurse and I am an expert in delivering expert healthcare to children." Or, "I am a pediatric nurse, and I am an expert in the special physical, emotional, and developmental healthcare needs of children."

Your turn. Define and claim your expertness:

_____
_____
_____
_____
_____
_____

## Informational Interviewing

Breathing life into your career can sometimes mean moving to another practice area. You may feel that you need the challenge and stimulation of a rapid learning curve or it may be that you've always dreamed of working in a particular practice area, but time seems to slip away. Whatever the reason, informational interviewing can speed the process and clear the way toward a smoother transition to another area.

Informational interviewing is a tool to gather the data or information to help you learn more about something. For instance, suppose you are interested in working in the OR. Informational interviewing is an excellent way to find out much more of what you need to know to learn about the OR, apply to the OR, and practice in the OR.

Here's what you would do. Find out the name of a respected nurse who works in the OR. Contact him or her and ask if you might have approximately a half-hour to ask some questions about practicing in the OR. Hint: Be appreciative of people's time and don't ask for more than one half-hour.

It might go something like this: "Hi, Tom. I'm thinking about transferring to the OR, and I'm wondering if you would be available for about a half-hour at your convenience to answer some of the questions I have about working in the OR. I'd appreciate any suggestions you might have."

Generally people are enthusiastic about answering questions for an informational interview. When it's time for the interview, make sure you are prompt and that you wrap up the questions and thank the interviewee for his or her time. It's also thoughtful to follow up with a written thank-you note, just as you would with a regular job interview.

Here are some questions you might ask during an informational interview:

- What do you think is the best preparation for working in the OR?
- What do you think is the best part of your practice? The worst?
- What educational preparation would you recommend?
- What is a typical day like for you?
- What do you think most nurses don't understand about working in the OR?

Informational interviewing is a great opportunity to get your feet wet in a different practice area without leaving your job. And it's a great way to find a mentor along the way!

## Networking

Networking is not for the business world anymore. Networking is found in every occupation and even in our social lives. Except for nurse executives, networking is usually not on the radar screen of most nurses, but it's an important tool to add to your list of acquired skills.

Networking is not all that mysterious. If you belong to a nursing organization and attend meetings – you're networking. You're meeting and greeting and exchanging information with colleagues you know and those you've just met.

And like most business protocol, networking does involve a sort of etiquette. Some important things to remember include:

- Decide what you want to accomplish at the event and make that a priority.

- Wear your nametag on your right shoulder. It makes it easier for the other person to read when you shake hands.

- Don't hang around the bar or the food. Mingle.

- It's sometimes helpful to have a prepared intro for yourself that will interest other people.

- Don't monopolize someone's time or attention. Chances are that person is trying to network as well.

- Don't hand out your business card to everyone.

- When someone hands you his business card, look at it carefully before putting it away. Some people consider it rude to toss a card in a folder or pocketbook without looking at it first.

- Try to listen more than you talk.

## Versatility in Nursing

There are few careers that have the versatility that nursing offers. Critical care, labor and delivery, pediatrics, OR, med/surg...the list goes on. And those are just the more conventional careers in nursing. The nursing profession has expanded into new areas as well – forensics, for example.

The point is, there is little chance of becoming bored in the nursing profession. You can always take your career to another practice area or even create a new practice area. Nurses today are practicing in administration, schools, laboratories, field tents, and on computers, to name just a few areas.

Whatever your interest, chances are you can match a nursing career to fit it. For example, you might be interested in research and could find professional happiness working as a nurse participating in clinical trials. Or you might be interested in solving crimes and could work as a nurse death investigator or forensics nurse. You might be loaded with persuasive skills and find success as a pharmaceutical sales manager or a nurse attorney. You might love the thrill of excitement and would be challenged by practicing as a flight nurse. You get the picture – nursing offers something for everyone.

So before you consider leaving the profession, ask yourself – Is there a better fit for my skills and passion in nursing? Would I be better suited and happier in another practice area?

Take time to journal. If there were no barriers to where and how I practice, what area of nursing would I like to try out?

_____

_____

_____

What are the barriers that I think are standing in my way of trying that practice area?

_____

_____

_____

_____

_____

If I'm really honest with myself, which barriers can be eliminated?

_____

_____

_____

_____

_____

"Adopt the following perspective – change brings opportunity," says Jane Kalagher, RN, MA, a coach who works with nurses at midlife. "Get into motion. Any movement opens doors – unexpected opportunities that you can't imagine!"

Jane recommends the following ideas to get momentum:

- Identify the top ten professional values that are important to you (i.e., leadership, contribution, assertiveness).
- Develop new skill sets and skill levels that will facilitate success.
- Take the time to explore multiple career possibilities.
- Explore and research your areas of interest.
- Create a crystal clear professional vision of what you want.
- Create a long-term and short-term plan to accomplish your vision.
- Don't settle. Don't let obstacles keep you from moving forward.
- Take action.

You have a life and a career that is waiting for you – and it's much bigger than you can ever imagine. You just need to understand who you are and what makes you unique, understand and appreciate your weaknesses and strengths, and finally, understand what success means to you. Go ahead now...reach for that STAR©!

# Resources and Bibliography

Covey, S. *First Things First*. Fireside; New York, NY:1995.

Rimm, S. *How Jane Won*. Crown Publishers; New York, NY:2001.

(Partial List)
Academy of Medical-Surgical Nurses. Available at: www.medsurgnurse.org.
Advance for Nurses. Available at: www.advanceweb.com.
Air & Surface Transport Nurses Association. Available at: www.astna.org.
American Academy of Ambulatory Nursing. Available at: www.aaacn.org.
American Academy of Nurse Practitioners. Available at: www.aanp.org.
American Association of Critical-Care Nurses. Available at: www.aacn.org.
American Association of Diabetes Educators. Available at: www.aadenet.org.
American Association of Legal Nurse Consultants. Available at:
www.aalnc.org.
American Association of Neuroscience Nurses. Available at: www.aann.org.
American Association of Nurse Anesthetists. Available at: www.aana.com.
American Association of Occupational Health Nurses. Available at:
www.aaohn.org.
American Association of Spinal Cord Nurses. Available at: www.aascin.org.
American Forensic Nurses. Available at: www.amrn.com.
American Holistic Nurses' Association. Available at: www.ahna.org.
American Long Term & Sub Acute Nurses Association. Available at:
www.alsna.com.
American Nephrology Nurses Association. Available at: www.annanurse.org.
American Nursing Informatics Association. Available at: www.ania.org.
American Psychiatric Nurses Association. Available at: www.apna.org.
American Radiological Nurses Association. Available at: www.arna.net.
American Society of Ophthalmic Registered Nurses. Available at:
http://webeye.ophth.uiowa.edu/asor.
American Society of Pain Management Nurses. Available at: www.aspmn.org.
American Society of PeriAnesthesia Nurses. Available at: www.aspan.org.
American Society of Plastic Surgical Nurses, Inc. Available at: www.aspsn.org.
Association for Professionals in Infection Control and Epidemiology, Inc.
Available at: www.apic.org.

Association of Nurses in AIDS Care. Available at: www.anacnet.org.
Association of Pediatric Oncology Nurses. Available at: www.apon.org.
Association of periOperative Registered Nurses. Available at: www.aorn.org.
Association of Rehabilitation Nurses. Available at: www.rehabnurse.org.
Association of Women's Health, Obstetric, and Neonatal Nurses. Available at: www.awhonn.org.

Case Management Society of America. Available at: www.cmsa.org.

Dermatology Nurses Association. Available at: www.dna.inurse.com.
Developmental Disabilities Nurses Association. Available at: www.ddna.org.

Emergency Nurses Association. Available at: www.ena.org.
Endocrine Nurses Society. Available at: www.endo-nurses.org.

Home Healthcare Nurses Association. Available at: www.hhna.org.
Hospice and Palliative Nurses Association. Available at: www.hpna.org.

Infusion Nurses Society. Available at: www.ins1.org.
International Association of Airline Nurses. Available at: (817) 963-1200.
International Nurses Society on Addictions. Available at: www.intnsa.org.
International Society of Nurses in Genetics. Available at: http://nursing.creighton.edu/isong.
International Transplant Nurses Society. Available at: www.itns.org.

National Association of Clinical Nurse Specialists. Available at: www.nacns.org.
National Association of Neonatal Nurses. Available at: www.nann.org.
National Association of Nurse Massage Therapists. Available at: www.nanmt.org.
National Association of Orthopaedic Nurses. Available at: http://naon.inurse.com.
National Association of School Nurses. Available at: www.nasn.org.
National Nursing Staff Development Organization. Available at: www.nnsdo.org.
Nurse Healers Professional Associations. Available at: www.therapeutic-touch.org.
Nursing Spectrum. Available at: www.nursingspectrum.com.

Oncology Nursing Society. Available at: www.ons.org.

Society for Vascular Nursing. Available at: www.svnnet.org.
Society of Gastroenterology Nurses and Associates. Available at: www.sgna.org.
Society of Otorhinolaryngology and Head-Neck Nurses, Inc. Available at: www.sohnnurse.com.
Society of Pediatric Nurses. Available at: www.pedsnurses.org.
Society of Urologic Nurses and Associates. Available at: www.suna.org.

Wound, Ostomy, and Continence Nurses Society. Available at: www.wocn.org.

# Chapter Seven

## Calling the Code

"There are two ways of meeting difficulties. You alter the difficulties or you alter yourself to meet them."

Elizabeth Barrett Browning

Sometimes things are just not fixable. Or at least they are not fixable in your lifetime. Thankfully, this doesn't happen all the time. Usually a miserable working environment is fixable or at least endurable. But for some of you reading this chapter, the end of the road for you is clear.

You're miserable on the job and you're in pain. You dread going to work everyday and your weekends seldom bring you respite from the anticipated dread of your next shift. You find yourself often daydreaming about quitting and walking away from it all.

There comes a tipping point where just one more thing will move you to that place where enough's enough and it's time to fish or cut bait. As much as that tipping point can bring a feeling of glorious relief that you can finally walk away from the source of your pain, still, there is some grieving for what you had and what you lost.

In this chapter, we'll look at managing the pain and making the decision to move on – whether it's to another practice area, another healthcare facility, or even leaving the nursing profession.

### Pain Management

It hurts. You studied long and hard for a career in nursing. You even grew up planning to be a nurse and converting the toy doctor bag, with the colorful stethoscope and the candy "medicine", into a nurse's satchel to treat your dolls and little brother. You just never thought it would come to this – a need to get some space between you and your childhood dreams and this profession.

There's no doubt that the nursing profession has a way of seeping into the very core of who you are. It's difficult to separate the nurse from who you are as a person, because so much of what you value in nursing – the healing and nurturing – are so much a part of who you are as a person. Yet, you know it's time to move on and leave a profession that has given you so much, yet wounded you at the same time.

Still, you know that nursing is a fabulous career with enormous satisfaction and opportunities for growth and learning. Few careers offer the versatility and an opportunity to make a difference that nursing provides.

So when is it time to move on? Unfortunately, there is no magic formula to tally what will unequivocally add up to your tipping point. Moving on is a personal decision and should be made after careful consideration.

Here are some reasons (some more common than others) for moving on:

- Toxic workplace environment
- Difficult or toxic coworker(s)
- Personal demands (moving, births, deaths, financial needs)
- Unsafe work environment
- Lack of support or leadership
- Boredom or lack of challenge
- Geographical distance (facility is too far from home)
- Lack of advancement opportunities

According to Sue Tobin, RN, CPCC, a life coach who specializes in working with nurses, it's important to name the discomfort that is showing up and if it has a physical manifestation (i.e., upset stomach, diarrhea, headaches, tense neck/shoulders, aching back). "Is that discomfort showing up as anger, resentment, frustration, fatigue?" asks Sue. "Do they feel melancholy, depressed, sad, lonely, isolated or callous in their nursing practice?"

Midlife coach Jane Kalagher says that nurses at midlife and midcareer often feel caught between a rock and a hard place. "The frustrations that arise from the healthcare system, coupled with the typical pattern of working for years in the same position or field, often leave the nurse feeling exhausted and passionless," says Jane. She recommends that before nurses leave the profession, they should "Stop, pause, and carefully identify their values and passions." Some of her questions below may be helpful:

- Do I feel stuck within my position? Within my particular field of nursing?

- Have my interests and passions changed? If so, what are they?

- What are my possibilities within the nursing profession?

- Am I willing to explore all the possibilities?

- What area and position might be an excellent match for me?

- What have I never considered?

When you are miserable at work, those feelings have a way of following you home and invading your personal life. The opposite is also true. If your personal life is miserable, those feelings can accompany you to work, too. So, you need to be clear on the originating source of your misery.

When trying to sort out your thoughts and feelings about whether you should leave your job or the nursing profession, it is helpful to make a pros and cons list to more accurately weigh the options.

List the pros and cons to leaving your job.

PROS                              CONS

_____        _____
_____        _____
_____        _____
_____        _____
_____        _____

Now, a simple pros and cons list won't definitively tell you which decision should be made. However, it is a tool to help you along the path toward a decision. You might also consider consulting a career coach, your employee assistance program (EAP), or a trusted and respected mentor to help you objectively sort the data and your feelings. Perhaps you might consider taking some time out from your position to gain some space and perspective. Or, perhaps your employer would consider allowing you to temporarily transfer to another practice area rather than lose a valued employee.

Take a moment to journal. Find a quiet place and allow yourself the luxury of thinking and reflecting alone to consider and weigh your options. Finish this sentence:

When I quiet myself and listen to my True North, it tells me to:

_____

_____

_____

Making the decision to leave nursing is not to be taken lightly. You studied hard, learned so much in the trenches, and have made such a difference to your patients and your colleagues. Exhaust every avenue before leaving the profession behind. But should you find that no other avenue exists for you, take good care of yourself and know that you'll be missed.

# For more information

Jane Kalagher, RN, MA, Coaching Resources
Website: www.coachingresources.com.
E-mail: jane@coachingresources.com

Sue Tobin, RN, CPCC. Coach for Nurses
Website: www.coach4nurses.com
E-mail: coachSueTobinRN@aol.com

# Chapter Eight

## Nurses' Notes

"Communication is a measurable asset."
Susan Sampsell

In the real estate world, the mantra is, "location, location, location." In the academic world, it is "publish or perish." In the nursing world, it is "if it isn't documented, it isn't done."

Every nurse has had the importance of documentation drilled into his or her head before leaving nursing school and hitting the floors. That speaks to the importance the healthcare community, and the legal system, puts on words.

Most nurses try their best to document what needs documenting, but we've been less successful documenting beyond a patient's chart and telling the story of nursing to the community. And the spoken word has not fared much better. According to results of the Woodhull Study on Nursing and the Media, nurses were cited only 4% of the time in more than 2,000 health-related articles (Woodhull, 1997).

Nurses have a story to tell and a message to share with the public. We know the public wants to hear from us – they trust nurses. In fact, nurses rank first as the most honest and ethical profession (Gallup Poll, 2003). Yet only a few nurses dare to write or speak. Let's take a look at the importance of writing and speaking about the nursing profession.

### The Power of Words

It's pretty clear in watching television news, prime-time shows, and the print media that nurses are missing in action in the media. Prime-time dramas, such as *ER* and similar medical shows, showcase physicians as the flagship story line and nurses as incidental to the healthcare drama. Nursing doesn't fare much better in the news media. Nurses are seldom shown as spokesperson for any healthcare event, even if it's a nursing story. If a nurse is shown as a spokesperson, he or she is seldom identified as a nurse and is identified instead

102

as a "hospital spokesperson." Pick up a magazine or newspaper and nurses are seldom quoted as expert authorities, though in many cases nurses would be a perfect fit.

Who better than nurses to speak to the healthcare issues and concerns of the average citizen? It's up to all of us to promote nursing and healthcare information by using the written and spoken word – in other words, writing and speaking.

Now before you start feeling faint from the mere thought of writing a healthcare article, or worse, standing before an audience to (gasp!) speak, remember that you are a nurse and you can do anything! What you do everyday in providing patient care is extraordinary and remarkable. You use critical thinking skills and triage what would cause most people in any other occupation to throw in the towel. Very few people can do what you do everyday. With that said, let's get you ready to face the world with a pen in one hand and a microphone in the other.

**Write What You Know**

You know your area of practice. You are an expert in your area of practice. You possess information that would benefit novice nurses or nurses outside your area of practice. Before you throw your hands up and protest that you can't write because you are a bedside nurse or a nurse that lacks 25 credentials after your name – you're not getting off that easy!

Nurses who practice at the bedside are the hands-down experts. You put theory into practice everyday. You know what works and what doesn't, and you have a human connection to your patients. You can't separate theory from the in-the-flesh patient in front you. Compared to what you do everyday, writing is a piece of cake.

Let me take the mystery out of writing for you. You do not have to be a great writer to write. Heck, you don't even need to be a great writer to be on the *New York Times* bestseller list! The truth is, there are very few great writers out there – probably a handful. The rest of the writers in the world have varying degrees of competency and skill. Writing is a skill that is developed with use, much like starting an IV. Some nurses are better at it than others, but certainly most nurses could improve their IV starts simply by doing them more often and brushing up on tried-and-true techniques.

Most nurses don't think they know anything worth writing about. But think about it, the public is thirsty for health information. Just look at the explosion of healthcare sites on the Internet. They are driven by the demand of the healthcare consumer. Nurses are in a perfect position to answer that demand.

A perfect example is Jerri Colonero, RN. Jerri had worked for years as a staff nurse in a labor and delivery unit. When managed care shortened the length of stay for new moms, Jerri felt frustrated by the volume of information she needed to give in so little time. So, Jerri decided to write a book (*With You and Your Baby All the Way*) for new parents. And she didn't let a lack of writing or publishing experience hold her back. Instead, she researched what she needed to know, used healthcare colleagues to review her work, and met with publishing success. Her book became unique among childcare books and quickly rose on the Amazon.com book list.

You can do the same thing. For instance, an ED nurse could write an article for the local newspaper on bike helmet safety. Or how about health prevention information on the flu? Or dressing a wound and when to seek the advice of a healthcare professional?

The OR nurse could write about what to expect when surgery is needed (patients seldom get this information from their physicians). Patients often don't understand what to expect when they are admitted and certainly have little understanding of what to expect when they are discharged. Or how about information about right-site surgery?

The psychiatric nurse (and especially the psychiatric advanced practice nurse) could write about managing mental illness at home, educate the public about some aspect of mental illness, and certainly inform the public that mental illness can be treated by a psychiatric APN who has prescriptive authority and can partner with the patient to navigate them through mental illness.

The pediatric nurse could write about childhood illnesses or injuries. How about croup and when to call your healthcare provider? Managing chickenpox? Head lice?

You get the picture. Every practice area provides an opportunity to educate the public about the nurse's role and what they need to know to keep them healthy, safe, and informed. Nurses do this everyday at the bedside, in schools, and in clinics. You just need to put it in writing.

The bottom line is, you figure out what you want to write and you write it.

Let's break it down:

1.  What am I going to write about? If you don't have much experience writing, it's probably best to write about what you already know, rather

than trying to bring yourself up to speed on a topic you know little about.

Terry is a school nurse who wants to write about handling respiratory distress in children. That's a good start. She knows what she wants to write about and has ample experience with respiratory distress in children and feels confident she can access any additional information she might need from nurse and physician colleagues. But now what?

2.  Narrow your focus. One of the biggest mistakes a novice writer makes is keeping the scope of the topic too big. This makes it difficult (and overwhelming!) to get your hands around the topic and cover it competently for your reader. So, when you have a topic, ask yourself, How can I break this down into a smaller components? Let's go back to Terry:

Terry is beginning to panic. Where should she begin? After all, there are so many causes of respiratory distress in children and she's noticed that most of the articles in her local newspaper on the op/ed (opinion/editorial) page are around 700 words or so. That's not enough room! Wait a minute, Terry thinks, what if I just write about asthma? And maybe narrow the focus even more to managing asthma at home.

3.  Brainstorm. Once you have settled on a topic and narrowed the focus of the topic enough, it's time to brainstorm. This is a simple technique that helps you collect and capture all the thoughts you have in your mind and write them down. Most of us are far too busy for our own good. This means our brains are cramped with billions of bits of information that we always think we'll be able to remember. The truth is, we often forget things because we're still cramming into our brains other thoughts and things to remember. By writing down all the thoughts you have about your topic, you are less likely to forget anything.

Terry takes 15 minutes to collect her thoughts about asthma. She doesn't bother to write complete sentences; she just wants to capture her thoughts before they are gone. Terry also doesn't bother censoring her thoughts. Just collect them, she thinks, and I'll delete stuff later. Better to have everything on the brainstorm list now and sort it out later. Her list includes: peak flow meters, assessing respiratory distress, signs and symptoms, common medications, proper use of inhalers and school nurses.

4.  The dreaded outline. We all remember learning about writing outlines in high school and feeling that it was a waste of time and effort. The outline has been much maligned and misunderstood. It is meant to be a tool that helps put your article together easily. If you spend some time doing your outline, the article can practically write itself. It's really simple. Take your brainstorm list and group similar ideas together. Then look at your groups of ideas and think about what order the groups should go in. Bingo! You have yourself an outline.

Terry looks at her brainstorm list and begins to group similar ideas together. She's not sure on the order yet, but here's part of her working outline:

I. Asthma
a) definition
b) incidence

II. Peak Flow Meters
a) different types of peak flow meters
b) how to use peak flow meters
c) importance of recording peak flow results

III. Role of School Nurse
a) parents partnering with school nurse to manage asthma
b) nurse partnering with healthcare provider
c) inhalers and peak flow meters in school

IV. Asthma Attack
a) school setting or at home
b) parent and healthcare provider contact info
c) assessing respiratory status
d) cold weather, illness, stress

5.  Know your audience. You know what you want to write and your outline is in working order. The next step is to have an understanding of who your audience is and what their understanding of your topic is.

If you understand who your audience is, you will then know how to write to them. For instance, if you write an article for the general public, you will need to use terminology that they understand – or define medical terminology. You will need to break down the information to a level that is understandable to someone outside the healthcare profession. Otherwise, what's the point? Or if you are writing an article for your specialty nursing journal, you will be writing for a like group of people who have a specialized grasp of the topic. You won't need to define simple terminology or concepts.

Terry's outline is complete. She wants to share her knowledge with the public and believes that her local newspaper op/ed page would be a good place to start. It's kind of like writing for my neighbors, she thinks. She realizes that she's going to break her terminology down to understandable terms and that perhaps her outline is too big. After all, she's going to need to chunk down the information. She decides to limit her outline to the handling of asthma in the school setting and just briefly touch on the growing incidence of asthma in the school-age population. She figures this will do two things – 1. educate the community (especially parents) about what they need to know about managing asthma in the school setting, and 2. educate the community about the expertise and knowledge base of the school nurse in managing asthma in the school setting.

6.  It's time to write. This is the fun part. Think back to high school composition. Your article should have three parts – the introduction, the body, and the conclusion. Think of it like a meal. The introduction is the appetizer – it whets the appetite of the reader and makes them excited about what's to follow. The body of the article is like the main course, where the reader has all the ingredients you want them to get from the article. And finally, the conclusion is the dessert, where the reader feels satisfied and completely full. Let's see how Terry does with each of them:

Terry understands that the three parts of her article need to be compelling so that people will take the time to read it. She knows that the introduction will have to be particularly compelling so that the people will want to read the article. She thinks about different ways she can start her article to pull the readers in. Hmmm...maybe I could ask a question of the readers about the incidence of asthma to make them feel like active participants in the article. Or maybe I could use an outstanding quote that relates to asthma. Humor? No, that doesn't seem appropriate for the topic. How about an interesting or surprising fact about asthma? Terry decides that she'll use the interesting or surprising fact to start her article.

For the body of the article, Terry decides she has to deliver the goods to the readers and fully answer and speak to the areas she decided to write about. She's taken the time to look at well-written topics on the op/ed page of her newspaper and has noted that the best articles are written using an active voice rather than a passive voice. So, rather than write about "the asthma support group that was started..." she'll write, "I started an asthma support group to..." She'll write in first person, rather than third person to make the article more alive and interesting.

Terry knows that she doesn't want her article to just drift off at the end. So, she'll make sure that her ending is as powerful and compelling as her introduction. She considers the same techniques for the introduction and decides that she'll end with a challenge to the readers to educate themselves about childhood asthma and voice their support of school nurses to their school systems, so that children with asthma can have the support they need to stay in the classroom – learning.

7. Avoid pretentious writing. We're so afraid of simple writing, yet simple writing is more understandable to the audience, and isn't that the whole point? It can be just as difficult to write simple and concise sentences. Here are some examples:

**Okay:** A modification of the original care plan was made by the staff nurse.

**Better:** The staff nurse modified the care plan.

**Okay:** The finalization of the program was brought about by the committee, but only after 10 hours of discussion had been conducted.

**Better:** The committee approved the plan after 10 hours of discussion.

**Okay:** The nurse manager **utilizes** a computerized scheduling system **in order** to provide a **very** equitable coverage of shifts.

**Better:** The nurse manager uses a computer-based scheduling system to provide equitable shift coverage.

8.  Someone once said that "words never cry out...but the author usually does." One of the most difficult things about writing is editing your work and then having an editor cut and slash some of the words you so painstakingly put onto paper. However, editing is meant to make your article the best it can be from an objective point of view. The author is often too close to the work to see the total picture with any perspective. Here are some tips for tightening your work before you send it off to the editor:

a) Edit ad nauseum! Read through your article over and over again. You will probably find some error each time you go through it. Common errors include spelling and grammatical mistakes, punctuation mistakes (i.e., no period at the end of a sentence), and extra words (i.e., See **the the** dog run).

b) Read it out loud. Sometimes when you read your article out loud, you may find that you trip over a mistake that you didn't see when you read the article to yourself.

c) Get a fresh view. Ask a colleague to read the article and see if it flows okay, if it makes sense, if you've missed anything, and so forth. For instance, Terry could ask a school nurse colleague to read it and then perhaps ask a nonnurse to read it.

d) Summarize each paragraph. This is a great tip if you've written an article and aren't sure if the flow from paragraph to paragraph makes sense. Here's what you do: Read each paragraph and in the left-hand margin, write one sentence summarizing the paragraph. Do this for every paragraph. Then go back and just read each sentence in the left-hand margin. The sentences should flow easily and make sense. If you feel yourself caught up by one sentence, it could be that the paragraph doesn't belong there and needs to be moved to a more appropriate place, or it doesn't belong in the article at all.

e) Out of sight, out of mind. Give yourself some time away from the article. Don't look at it for a day or two. Then go back and read it again. This will give you the opportunity to get some distance and perspective on the article so you can look at it once more with fresh eyes.

f) So what? Ask yourself, What does this mean to the reader? If you can answer that question with a few sentences, you probably have a pretty focused article. If it takes more than that to answer the question – or worse, you can't answer the question – chances are the article is not focused enough.

So, there you have it. Some basic tips for writing your article. Keep in mind that you should think about recycling your article. For instance, Terry could write her article on asthma for her professional school nurse journal, then she could re-write it for a nursing magazine geared for all nurses, then she could re-write it for a lay publication – local newspaper, parenting magazines, and so forth. Each audience, or readership, has a different level of understanding, and Terry would need to be mindful of the terminology and understanding the topic and write to that level.

Terry submitted her article to the op/ed editor of her local newspaper and was thrilled to see it appear several weeks later. Parents congratulated and thanked her for writing such an informative article, and people around town stopped her in the grocery store to talk about the article. Terry was surprised by the impact of writing one article and the difference it made on her self-esteem. So she decided to re-write the article for a parenting magazine. She spoke with a neighbor, a writer, who offered these suggestions:

- Study the writers' guidelines. Her neighbor explained that most publications have writing guidelines that are essentially the rules of the road for submitting an article. He suggested that she go to the local library or the bookstore and take a look at *The Writer's Market*, which is a book published annually that lists magazines, the name of the editor, the types of articles they are looking for, payments for articles, writing guideline information, and more. Terry's neighbor told her that ignoring the editor's preferred guidelines was a sure way to get rejected.

- Familiarize yourself with the magazine. If you are submitting an article to a particular magazine, make sure that you know what type of articles they do publish and what topics they have recently covered. If Terry submits an awesome article on asthma to the parenting magazine, but

110

the editor just published an article on that topic a month ago, the article will be rejected.

- Make your audition count. Terry's neighbor explained that most editors require a query letter before an article is sent in. *The Writer's Market* is a good place to find out if a query letter is required. He explained to Terry that a query letter is a one-page letter that explains what Terry plans to write on, why she's qualified to write it, and why the editor's readership would be interested in reading it. Terry's neighbor also told her that the query letter should be error-free and grammatically perfect, compelling, and as well written as Terry can make it. "It's your audition," said her neighbor.

- Meet that deadline. If Terry's query letter is well received and the editor asks her to write the article, she better meet that editor's deadline. If not, she can forget having the article published or ever working with that editor again.

- Remember to keep a copy. Terry's neighbor shared a litany of nightmares of novice writers who sent off their article (hardcopy and disk), but forgot to save the article for themselves. It usually only happens once!

Now it's your turn. Brainstorm some ideas of topics you could write about. Remember that you are an expert in your area of practice. What healthcare information can you share with your community? Don't censor your thoughts; just jot them down.

_____

_____

_____

_____

_____

_____

Read through your topics. Is there a topic that jumps out at you or one that makes you more excited than the others? Go with your feelings and pick that topic. It's easier and more enjoyable to go with a topic that excites you or that you feel strongly about. You're busy enough without picking a topic that you dread or that holds no interest for you. Use this as an opportunity to learn even more about something you enjoy.

## Step Up to the Microphone

Now that you've successfully finished your first article – or you're well on your way, it's time to look at another way nurses can share health information and educate the public about nursing – public speaking.

Now before you start to hyperventilate, remember that compared to what you do everyday in your practice, writing and public speaking is a piece of cake. And just like writing, you don't need to be a great speaker or a charismatic speaker. You need to be competent. You just need to have a message and deliver it cleanly and in an understandable way. Think of all the seminars or speeches you have heard over the years, some of them by highly educated and acclaimed individuals. But most of them were probably not compelling speakers. They may have had a message, but little clue how to deliver it to the audience. Think of the times that you've sat in an audience and felt as if your eyelids had ten-pound weights on them as you sat pinching yourself to stay awake. You can do better than that!

Nurses often complain that no one understands what they bring to the healthcare table. Speaking is an opportunity to change that. So take a deep breath, step up to the microphone, and let your voice be heard. Here's how to get started:

1. Decide on your objective. What do you want to speak about and what do you want your audience to get from your presentation? Remember, you want to be focused, just like in your writing, and not tackle a topic that's too big.

2. Brainstorm. Capture all the ideas you have about the topic on paper. Now is not the time to edit your thoughts. Brainstorming should be done as quickly as you can so that your critical mind can't interfere.

3. You know what's next. Sort the ideas in your brainstorming list and create like or similar groups. Then decide the order of each group to create your outline.

4. The presentation should be set up just like your article – with an introduction, body, and conclusion. And just like the article, you want to pull your audience in right away with your introduction, with either an interesting quote, anecdotal story, interesting or surprising fact, a challenge, or humor (be careful!).

5. Pick three to four points that you will address, no more. Any more than that is often difficult for the audience to remember.

6. Use visuals to help deliver your message, but don't overdo it or get beyond your technological capability. It's been said that the average person needs to hear something seven to fifteen times before he or she gets the message. Many parents can attest to that! So use your visuals to support and reinforce the points you want your audience to walk away with. Most people are visual learners. We tend to only remember 10% of what we hear, but we remember more than 50% of what we hear and see (Axtell,1992).

7. In your presentation, tell the audience what you're going to tell them, then tell them, and then tell them what you told them! Think of it like a television sports show. The pregame show is when the sportscasters talk about what is going to happen, and then during the actual sporting event they tell you what you're seeing. During the postgame show the sportscasters then tell you what you just saw.

8. Make your conclusion compelling and memorable. Don't just drift off with an apologetic, "Well, that's all I have to say. Thank you." End your speech with an inspiring quote that relates to your topic. Or challenge your audience to make a difference with your subject matter. You could also end with a patient story that dramatizes and supports your points.

9. Make eye contact. People who have to give presentations are often so unnerved that they avoid eye contact. What a mistake. Making eye contact with your audience is a way to project and convey your power, and it's a way to connect with the audience so that they listen to you and consider what you're saying. And isn't that the whole point? The trick is to make sure that you know your presentation so well that you can look up (if you're reading or referring to notes), look to the left and

113

make eye contact, then look to the center, then look to your right and make eye contact, without losing your spot or your concentration.

10. Which brings me to, rehearse, rehearse, rehearse. Invite a colleague to listen to you rehearse. Does the flow seem okay? Does he or she get your points? Are there any words or phrases that you trip over or that sound awkward? Time yourself. If you've been given 20 minutes to give a speech, make sure you don't run over.

You're finally ready to give that speech. Here are some last words of advice to get you off to a good start. You'll need to dress the part, which means dressing professionally and a little dressier than you expect your audience will be; usually a beautiful suit (pantsuit is fine for women), polished shoes (low heel is best for women). Be sure the outfit is comfortable. You want to feel and look great. Think about the image you want to covey. Certainly, you want to convey your personal power and that you are an expert. Colors that typically demonstrate power are red (the ultimate color of power) and black. Navy blue usually signifies sincerity (think of all the male politicians who campaign wearing their sincere navy suit with a red tie to convey power.) Yellow is a great color because the eye is attracted to it, and it's associated with learning, think – school bus. Women should avoid jangling jewelry that could be distracting if picked up by a microphone.

You look great! You've rehearsed. All that's missing is your confidence. Think about this: Giving this speech will change you in ways you can't imagine because it's all about risk and believing in yourself. You can do it. You can take a leap into the unknown abyss and push the envelope of who you thought you were. You are bigger than you can ever imagine. Giving a speech is all about owning your fear – instead of letting your fear own you. It's important to realize that you can never really get rid of your fear once and for all, but you can be the one who controls it. And giving a speech is one way to own your own power and to acknowledge to the world, and yourself, that you have something worthwhile to say.

Visualize yourself giving your speech and the audience enthusiastically clapping. (See chapter four for more about visualization). See their smiling faces in your mind. Hear the sound of loud clapping. Feel the pride in your body as you accept and acknowledge the applause. Visualize every night before you go to bed and during the day. Then again, visualize it an hour before the presentation and then right before you get up to speak. Then before you speak, take a moment to relax your body, take a deep breath, smile, and speak.

114

Author Janet Stone wrote about women and public speaking, "Almost all of us are born speakers; we had to be taught to sit down and shut up." (Strone & Bachner, 1994).

It's time you stand up and speak.

# Resources and Bibliography

Axtell, R. *Do's and Taboos of Public Speaking*. John Wiley & Sons, New York, NY:1992.

Colonero, J. *With You and Your Baby All the Way: Complete Guide to Pregnancy, Childbirth, Recovery, and Baby Care*. Bull Publishing:1998.

Drummond, ME. *Fearless and Flawless Public Speaking with Power, Polish, and Pizazz*. Pfeiffer, Inc. Toronto:1993.

Gallup Poll. Public rates nursing as most honest and ethical profession. Available at: www.gallup.com.

Goldberg, N. *Writing Down the Bones*. Shambhala Publications, Boston, MA:1986

Stone, J and Bachner, J. *Speaking Up: A Book for Every Woman Who Talks*. Carroll & Graff, New York, NY:1977, 1994.

Toastmasters International. Available at: www.toastmasters.org.

Ueland, B. *If You Want to Write*. Graywolf Press; St. Paul, MN:1938, 1983, 1987.

Woodhull Study on Nursing and Media. Commissioned by Sigma Theta Tau International, funded by Robert Wood Johnson Foundation, and conducted by University of Rochester School of Nursing. Available at: www.stti.org.

# Chapter Nine

# A Nurse Is a Nurse Is a Nurse

"Power is strength and the ability to see yourself through your own eyes and not through the eyes of another. It is being able to place a circle of power at your own feet and not take power from someone else's circle."

Lynn V. Andrews

Pick up a magazine, tabloid, newspaper, or watch tabloid/entertainment television, and you'll see that perception or image is a big industry. Celebrities spend vast amounts of money and time paying image consultants for a reason. Developing the right image is like money in the bank.

What's image got to do with you – a nurse? Everything. We know that nurses have an image of being trustworthy and hardworking. But the profession also has an image of being handmaidens to physicians, sex symbols, or battleaxes.

## Image

Does your image project who you are and who you want to become? In other words, if your ambition includes becoming a nurse manager on your unit, does your image project someone who could walk into that position?

At this point you may be saying, "Listen, I'm qualified to become a nurse manager because of the knowledge base I have and the leadership skills I've developed. Why do I have to look the part, too?"

Here's why. Healthcare is a business, in part run by business people. The business message, spoken or implied, that filters down the ladder is professionalism. Professionalism is not new in the nursing world, but how it is interpreted by the business end of healthcare is new. To move into the position you want, you have to have the skills and look the part.

Looking the part involves more than just the clothes you wear. It also involves learning the skills for the new role, speaking the language of that culture, and observing the unspoken rules of that culture.

Let's look at an example.

Mark is a skilled and highly regarded med/surg nurse. He's worked on the unit for seven years and has proven his mettle time and again. He usually wears scrubs and sneakers, and he's often called a big teddy bear because of his scruffy beard and hair that is often in need of a haircut. Mark loves med/surg, but he feels he's ready to move on to a different type of challenge. A nurse manager position has opened and he wants to apply for it.

Now if Mark is smart, he'll realize that he may have the qualifications necessary for the job, but he might not (in the eyes of the interviewers) have the image they are looking for. What are some things that Mark could do to better his chances for getting that nurse manager position?

- Think about his physical image for the interview. Get a professional haircut and trim his beard; wear a business suit, polished shoes, and a conservative tie.

- Leave the easy-going, back-slapping Mark outside the interview door. Project a professional and business-like demeanor that will allow the interviewers to easily picture him in the nurse manager role.

- Make an appointment to speak with one or more nurse managers he admires. What do they recommend he do to improve his chances of getting the position? What areas do they see lacking in him that he could improve on and be ready to address during the interview?

- Think about the interview from the perspective of the interviewers and those above them. If he were in their position, would he look favorably on him?

According to Lori Johnson, a certified image consultant and owner of Your Best Image, 55% of your influence upon others is based on your image or appearance. And you have less than 30 seconds to make a positive first impression. So whether you like it or not, people are making a decision about you based on the image you are projecting. Put your best foot forward. Here's some advice from Lori:

**Suit basics for men and women**

- Never have more than three patterns in a suit, shirt, or tie

118

- If you can afford only one suit, in most cases the best choice is a solid navy blue. Make sure that the lining is the same color tone. In most cases, brown is not a good choice.
- Keep skirt lengths no shorter than one inch above knee.
- The key to looking good is a good fit.

## Women

- Avoid revealing blouses
- Avoid dangling earrings. Earrings that dangle below the earlobe are distracting and can cause the face to be drawn down and look tired.
- If you can hear it, don't wear it. No bangle bracelets or tinkling earrings.
- Shoe colors should be same color value, or darker, than hemline. Basic leather pumps are best.

## Men

- White or off-white shirt is best. A small stripe in shirt is okay.
- Top button of the shirt should be buttoned under tie. If you can't put two fingers in your collar when buttoned, the shirt is too small.
- Tie should be current, but not trendy, and made of silk only. A safe width for a tie is three inches.

Developing a professional image to move your career forward doesn't have to be difficult. But it is a process. "Paying attention to and improving your total image will help you gain self-confidence and increase your self-esteem," says Lori. "It will increase your chances for success in everything you do."

## What Kind of Nurse Are You?

"Yeah, yeah, yeah," you say. "I'm happy at the bedside and I don't ever see myself applying for a nurse manager position. So what's this image thing got to do with me?"

Glad you asked. If you aren't perfectly happy with the image that nursing has in the public or the media or even where you work – then image has everything to do with you. There's an old saying, "If a tree falls in the forest but no one hears it, does it make a sound?" The answer is obvious.

However, if nurses don't tell people what they do, they are essentially practicing without making a sound. So the image you project in your practice influences the image your patients, their families, and your institution have about nursing. Like another old saying goes, "If you're not part of the solution, you're part of the problem."

Nurses need to be change agents. For instance, if you are a school nurse, you might be frustrated by school administrators who seem to not value your role or what you bring to the educational system. You may feel that you are just banging your head against the proverbial wall when you tell them the sheer volume of the students you care for everyday overwhelms you.

Consider that you might be talking to the wrong people. Who really holds the power in the school system? It's the parents! As a school nurse change agent, you might consider educating the parents about the number of students you care for and why it's important. Don't say you see "a lot" of students; give them statistics. When the parents truly understand what you do and how you impact their children, then the parents will drive the necessary changes. Bottom line – the school administration answers to the parents.

If you are satisfied with spending your career at the bedside (a perfectly admirable ambition), then you might consider striving to be the best nurse at the bedside; a bedside nurse with obvious leadership skills, and a bedside nurse who understands the impact and value of what you bring to the profession.

To do that, you must understand who you are as a person and a nurse. Let's get an idea of who you are. Remember that there is no right or wrong answer, it's just how and who you are. Some people are better at very detailed things (think accountants) while others are big picture people – they like to look at the overall picture (think visionary). Neither style is better than the other, and each style is an important part of the team. To think of it another way, if you're a big picture person, you might have a great idea for a program that would improve patient outcomes, while the detail person could take that idea and tie up all the loose ends to make the idea a reality.

Are you a detail person or a big picture person? How do you know?

_____

_____

_____

_____

Some people find they are most comfortable as members of a team. Other people are better at bringing a group of diverse people together as a team. The team player and the team builder bring different skills to the table. The team player is satisfied to fade into the background for the sake of the greater good, and compromise is a word that comes to the forefront. On the other hand, the team builder has to be able to persuade people to come together as one unit. The team builder has an idea of how the team should look and molds the team.

Are you a team player or a team builder? How do you know?

_____

_____

_____

_____

   Some people are quiet and prefer to be alone or in small groups. These people often find larger groups draining. Other people are more outgoing and prefer being around people. Large groups jumpstart their energy. Quiet people, or introverts, often are the type of people who delve more deeply into things and can bring vast amounts of insight to a situation. Outgoing people, or extroverts, often bring more energy to a situation and more easily connect with members of a group.

Are you an introvert or extrovert? How do you know?

_____

_____

_____

_____

What did you learn about yourself? Do you see how who you are is a part of what you are? How so? How does this show up in your practice?

_____

_____

_____

_____

_____

_____

   Understanding who you are provides insight into why you might feel more comfortable in a particular situation and uncomfortable in another situation. For instance, if you are more comfortable as a team player you might find a nurse manager role uncomfortable, since that's a role that calls for team building. The important message, however, is to understand that wherever you feel comfortable in your practice, you are still in a leadership position.

Business guru and author Stephen Covey has said that we are all leaders. The only difference is that we have a different circle of influence or audience (Covey, 1996). The VP of nursing at your facility has a larger circle of influence than you might, but you are both leaders. You can lead from anywhere you practice. As a member of the team, you can be a leader, influencing team members with your expertise and desire to make patients central to everything you do. You can influence your patients and their families with your body of knowledge and your willingness to guide them through their hospital experience. You can even influence those who hold positions above you or in meetings by sharing your insights and thoughts in a cogent and decisive manner. You can influence your community by sharing your healthcare expertise in different forums – PTA, career day at a local school, town meetings, and so forth.

You have the power to influence far beyond what you believe to be your circle. You just have to step up to the plate.

Let's look at some qualities of leadership:

- Accepting and understanding that you are a leader. If you do accept and understand that you are a leader, it will help make your actions more thoughtful.

- Be passionate. The most powerful leaders have a charisma about them, which is often fueled by the passion they feel about what they do.

- Be a risk taker. All leaders understand that there will be times when they have to put their money where their mouth is or step out on to that proverbial limb.

- Be guided by a value-based inner compass. A good leader is someone who isn't guided by how other people say it should be. Ignoring our inner values can come at a steep price. As James Champy and Nitin Nohria write in their book, *The Arc of Ambition*, "If morality seems expensive, consider the higher cost of immorality" (Champy, Nohria, 2000).

- Let go of the need to please. Pleasing others is not how a good leader judges him or herself.

## The Media

Speaking in public, writing, and developing a leadership image may sometimes mean that you find yourself in the media's crosshairs. This can be a good thing. Nurses should certainly consider how they can get the attention of the media to make nursing more visible.

Usually the public relations department of your institution handles the media. However, there may be a time when you are contacted directly to answer a question or to be interviewed, and you should be prepared to present a polished and informed image. (For more information on public speaking, see chapter eight)

Here are some things to consider:

- Know your message. When the media contacts you, take a few moments to collect your thoughts and consider exactly what message you want to deliver. You might find it helpful to have it written in front of you so you can bring the attention back to that message if the interview seems to veer in another direction.

- Think and speak in sound bites. A reporter is always listening for that magical quote that will look good in print and attract the attention of the readers. Pay attention to how politicians speak. They often deliver their message in short, powerful sentences (in other words, sound bites) that they know the voters will remember and the press will report in their coverage. Think about what your message is and turn it into a sound bite.

- Keep the reporter's perspective in mind. The reporter has a mission – to write an interesting article that will catch the attention of the readers and the boss! In addition, the reporter has a firm deadline that must be met. If you can give great sound bites in a timely manner, you've won a friend for life. Okay, maybe not a friend, but a reporter who may be receptive to future interviews.

- Understand who the ultimate audience is. When you are being interviewed, the reporter is not your audience – the public (i.e., readership or listening audience) is. Deliver your message so the audience understands it.

- Keep your cool. Sometimes reporters want to get the story behind the story – or the scoop. This will be the opposite of what you want. Keep your cool and remember that nothing is off the record. Do not say anything that you would not want to see in print. If you don't have an answer, you can say, "I don't know." If you like, you can offer to get back to the reporter with an answer or just leave it at that. Don't say, "No comment," as it makes you sound like you are hiding something. Sometimes reporters use provocative questions that are meant to get a rise out of the interviewee, or they try to put words in your mouth. Don't let them. Stop them immediately – politely – and correct them. Then repeat your message. Stay calm and don't let the reporter shake you up.

## Body Language

We communicate beyond our words and actions. It's been said that body language is 55% of any message we communicates (Drummond, 1993). Make sure that the message you convey through your words is matched by your body language. For instance, think about when you give a presentation. Don't for a minute think that you are judged only when you are up at the podium. The audience is passing judgment (or evaluating you) as soon as they see you, even while you are waiting to speak.

Maureen and her colleagues had to give a presentation to the school committee and the parents. Although only Maureen was scheduled to speak, she and her colleagues understood that the audience and the committee would be evaluating them the moment they walked in the door and waited their turn to do the presentation. They made sure their demeanor was professional at all times and that they did not appear nervous. When Maureen finished her presentation, they politely clapped and resisted every urge to "high-five" her because they knew they were still being sized up. The last thing they wanted was for the parents in the audience or the school committee to think that giving a presentation was a stretch for them.

During the presentation, Maureen remembered everything she had read about using body language to her advantage. Afraid that she would fidget with her hands, she placed her index fingers to her thumbs to stop her hands from shaking. She discovered that it immediately made her feel more relaxed. When she wanted to emphasize something, she imitated the "steeple" gesture that politicians use so often – placing her fingertips to fingertips with palms apart and fingers pointed upward. And she tried to own the space she was in by avoiding the fig leaf position where hands are clasped in front of the groin area. She knew that would make her look tentative and unsure of herself. Maureen took a few opportunities to step away from the podium and increase her physical space – thereby looking more authoritative and powerful. She understood that powerful people take up space, while unsure people shrink in their space (Josefowitz, 1990).

For Maureen, understanding how her image was received was an important part of making sure that the message received by the audience was the message she intended to send.

What message are you sending?

# Resources and Bibliography

Association of Image Consultants International. Available at: www.aici.org

Career/family information. Available at: www.BlueSuitMom.com.

Champy, J and Nohria, N. *The Arc of Ambition*. Perseus Books:2000.

Covey, S. *First Things First*. Fireside. New York,NY:1995.

Image consultant. Lori Johnson, Your Best Image. Website: www.yourbestimagepid.com. E-mail: lori@yourbestimagepid.com

Josefowitz, N. *Paths to Power*. Addison Wesley:1990.

Rimm, S. *How Jane Won: 55 Successful Women Share How They Grew from Ordinary Girls to Extraordinary Women*. Crown. New York, NY:2001.

Sample, S. *The Contrarian's Guide to Leadership*. Jossey-Boss:2002.

# Chapter Ten

# Positive Outcomes

"It takes as much energy to wish as it does to plan."
Eleanor Roosevelt

Much of this book has looked at developing a relationship with yourself again and figuring out who and what you are. It's difficult to figure out what you want if you aren't really sure who you are, what your strengths and skills are, and what is important and meaningful to you.

Hopefully, you are much closer to understanding yourself a bit better and ready to put your hopes and dreams into action. You've learned some valuable tools in this book – informational interviewing, setting those all-important boundaries, defining success on your terms, and much more. You now stand ready to charge down the path toward success. But wait a second – what do I do next, you ask? Sure, I have a better idea of what I want, but how do I get from here to there?

Remember, action steps, by putting one foot in front of the other. So let's get to it!

## Achievable Goals

You need to set achievable goals, and you need to understand what outcome you want. Goals are different from your dreams and your visions. Your dreams and visions are feeling-based and represent the big picture. Goals are the tangible parts that make up your dreams and visions.

Let's differentiate between goals and visions or dreams. You might have a dream or vision of finally losing those last 15 pounds. That's the picture you hold in your mind, and you have feelings attached to it – you may be miserable and disappointed in yourself now, but imagining yourself 15 pounds lighter makes you feel happy. You imagine that achieving that goal will make you feel proud. Your goal, on the other hand, is losing those last 15 pounds, but it's made up of the nitty-gritty steps that will make the vision a reality. Some of those steps may include walking four miles a day, decreasing your calorie intake by cutting out snacks, taking the stairs rather than an elevator, and

127

keeping a motivational journal. Setting achievable goals can move your career forward.

"Recall experiences that have really jazzed you up in your career," recommends Sue Tobin, RN, CPCC, a life coach who works with nurses. "What were you doing (task vs. talk), who were you with (alone or with patient or colleague). Were you learning, teaching, moving fast, counseling, investigating?" Understanding the specific aspects of those experiences can help you sort out what you need to feel jazzed up about your career again. Do you prefer doing tasks or interacting with a person? Do you prefer to work alone or does collaborating with colleagues jazz you? By asking the right questions, you can set your goal and put the action steps in place to move toward that goal.

According to Sue, written goals are an important component of measuring the nurse's journey of fulfillment through coaching. "Goals must be SMART. That is Specific, Measurable, Achievable, Realistic, and Time-determined tasks the nurse commits to," says Sue. "We all know nurses are reluctant to nurture themselves or take credit for achievement. These SMART goals are benchmarks to keep the nurse accountable to her commitment of personal and professional growth and development."

An important thing to remember is that you are allowed to change your goals and your visions if they no longer support you. You are allowed to change your mind! If your goal is to go back to school and become a nurse midwife, but you discover that your vision was not what you thought it was – you can change your mind. You always have a choice. As the old saying goes, if the shoes don't fit...don't wear them!

Another thing to keep in mind is that working toward your vision and your goals should be moving you closer to what you want and should be moving you to a happier place. If your vision and goals are not doing this, maybe you are holding a vision that is not really yours. If you're in tune with your values, you'll usually have a better sense of your vision and your goals.

Nancy is an OR nurse, but wants to move toward a nurse executive position. She enjoys patient care, but feels most fulfilled when she's problem solving or managing. Nancy has a solid understanding of her strengths and believes they are best suited for an executive position. When Nancy imagines her vision as a nurse executive, she sees herself as happy and fulfilled, leading the nursing staff, and providing an environment that supports nurses and patient care. Nancy writes down her vision: To be a nurse executive. Then she lists her goal: To move to a nurse executive position.

Finally, Nancy lists her action plan. Some of them include:

1. Complete an MBA program
2. Find a nurse executive mentor
3. Join a nursing organization that promotes nurse leadership
4. Look for opportunities to take a leadership role
5. Take a public speaking course

Each of the action steps that Nancy listed could be broken down further to make them more manageable and more easily achieved. For instance, here's how Nancy might break down the steps to an MBA degree:

1. Complete an MBA program
   a) research different MBA programs in the area
   b) call for a course catalog
   c) make an appointment with a college representative
   d) get my college transcripts and references in order

Accomplishing one action step will motivate Nancy and fuel her efforts to continue. So it's important that she set manageable, achievable, and realistic goals and action steps.

It's your turn. In chapter four you wrote down the vision you hold for yourself and how and when you will know when you've achieved it. It's time to take that vision and develop the goal and action steps that will make it a reality.

The vision I hold for myself is:

_____

_____

_____

_____

_____

Now list the steps (large and small) that you can take to make that vision come true for you.

Step 1:

_____

_____

Step 2:

_____

_____

Step 3:

_____

_____

Step 4:

_____

_____

It's important to make your goals achievable and realistic, otherwise, you'll become frustrated and stuck. Break the steps down as small as you can. Even a simple step such as making a phone call will generate a surge of positive energy that will give you the momentum to move to the next step. And that's what you want to create – momentum to carry you forward.

After you have listed every step you can think of, go back and date each step. In other words, by what date can you complete each one? When you've successfully completed one step, use that momentum and move to the next.

Don't get hung up and detoured by obstacles you place in your path. Many people resist following a vision or dream because they believe they are too old. "I'll be 55-years-old before I complete that degree!"

The truth is, you'll be 55-years-old one way or the other. You might as well arrive at that age having successfully completed a goal, rather than wistfully mourning what could have been. Ask yourself, How will I fell when I've achieved that goal? And how will I fell if I don't?"

Life is precious and you deserve to run at life full force. As long as you're still breathing, go after your dream. You know that your nursing practice gives you an inside view of the fragility of life. You deserve this. There is so much you need and want to accomplish. Push, move around, and go through any obstacles in your way. Don't chase old age...make it wait for you!

# Parting Thoughts

"It is not easy to find happiness in ourselves, and it is not possible to find it elsewhere."
Agnes Repplier

All journeys must come to an end, and this is no exception. You've covered a lot of territory and hopefully discovered many new and wonderful things about yourself. But remember, life is a constant journey and you have so much more to discover.

There are plenty of tools and strategies in this book that will move you toward what you want and away from what you don't want. But tools and strategies aside, please remember that the answers you are looking for are already inside you. You have the power to be the nurse you want to be and the person you want to be. You just have to ask yourself the right questions. Because it's the provocative questions that we ask ourselves that reveal who we are and how we can be the best we can be.

To give you an example: I worked with a nurse client who achieved great success in her career and had a happy family life, yet she was not happy. She told me that she felt empty. Coaching her involved helping her clear up the clutter and tolerations in her life and prioritizing her values and needs. But the essence of what she wanted was inside her, she was just too busy to see it. In her admirable journey of acquiring multiple academic degrees, moving up the ladder, and raising a family she had lost touch with who she was as a person. She forgot how to be happy.

I reminded her that happiness is not a destination; it's a choice we make at every juncture of our life. For her, "finding" happiness meant carving time out of her day – every day – to slow down enough to recognize, appreciate, and savor all the little moments in her day that made her happy or fulfilled. And also carve out time each day to do one little thing that made her happy. As any elderly person will tell you – happiness is in all the little moments we savor that will never come again.

Don't waste a moment. Don't be afraid to take a risk in your career. Give a presentation, write an article, or chair a committee. Life is constantly moving along and windows of opportunity are always opening and closing all around you. If you play it too safe and live in your comfort zone, those windows will slam shut before you get up the courage to take a chance. Don't get hung up on the idea that you must be perfect before you move forward. Because the truth is, you will never be perfect!

Relinquish the hold that perfection has on you – whether you use the pursuit of perfection as a means to an end or an excuse not to try. Human beings are not wired to be perfect. Allow yourself to be good enough, and move forward.

Keep your nursing career fresh. Sometimes the temptation for nurses who are busy raising families and working part-time is to forget that they are the managers of their career. Just because you practice part-time doesn't mean you shouldn't be invested in your career. Staying current, learning new skills, and managing your career will keep it fresh for you and broaden your options. There aren't many careers that allow the employee to jump from full-time to part-time to per diem to full-time again.

Educate your patients and the public about what you do as a nurse. One of my goals in writing this book is to help nurses' shore up their inner strength and claim their power and then move collectively to improve the image of the profession. You see, I don't think it's possible for the image of nursing to improve if the profession is made up of nurses who don't claim their individual power. The strength of a group is only as strong as the strength of each individual.

Finally, consider that we are never finished. We continue to grow, change, and learn until our last moment on earth. When you are elderly and nearing the end of your life, what regrets will you have? What might you have accomplished? What will you leave unfinished? If we're lucky and we strive to grow, change, and learn we will look back on our lives with fewer regrets and with more fulfilling moments to savor.

To that end, you might think about hiring a coach who can motivate you to continue along the path of success and fulfillment in your personal and professional life. Or consider gathering a group of nurse colleagues who wish to be coached together.

It is my sincerest hope that within these pages you found what you needed to jumpstart your career and the success and balance that you seek. I would love to hear how this book has helped you. To share your thoughts and comments, please e-mail me at coachborgatti@aol.com.

Printed in the United States
47425LVS00005B/352